Pain Relie

Pain Relief in the Orofacial Regions

Jens Kølsen Petersen

Associate Professor,
Department of Oral and Maxillofacial Surgery,
Royal Dental College,
Aarhus,
Denmark

Peter Milgrom

Professor,
Department of Dental Public Health Sciences,
School of Dentistry
Adjunct Professor,
Department of Health Services,
School of Public Health and Community Medicine,
Director, Dental Fears Research Clinic,
University of Washington, Seattle, Washington, USA

Munksgaard

Contents

Preface

Pain always has been with man, and man forever has tried to remove it. Because pain is a complex and integrated function of the human body, it is impossible to remove all types of pain at all times. Many dental patients seek help because they suffer from pain. Many expect the modern dental team to render them free from their suffering. If the dental team fails to relieve them from this pain, patients leave unhappy and bitter. Relieving pain is, of course, no simple matter. The orofacial regions are complex, as they consist of many different tissues with different functions, are richly innervated and vascularized, and project afferent sensations to the brain, where they are dispersed over a large area compared with the input from the rest of the body. The brain, in turn, gives high priority to orofacial sensations. It is, therefore, important that the members of the dental team be knowledgeable about pain mechanisms and pain treatment in these regions.

It is the authors' hope that this book can offer some insight into complex problem of dental pain and point to some solutions that might benefit our patients.

Jens Kølsen Petersen
Peter Milgrom

Acknowledgement

I would like to express my appreciation to colleagues Ross Beirne, Louis Fiset, Tracy Getz, and Philip Weinstein for advice on various aspects of this text. In addition I would like to indicate my sincere thanks to many patients in the Dental Fears Research Clinic at the University of Washington for allowing me to learn to know them in caring for their problem.

Finally, a note of appreciation is due to Lori Starrs at the University of Washington who edited the manuscript, and to Peter Egyedi at the National University of Singapore who read the entire manuscript and offered valuable suggestions.

Peter Milgrom

Introduction

Definition of pain

Pain is difficult to define. Most people think of pain as unpleasant and useless, and attempt to rid themselves of the pain they experience. Why, one might speculate, is living tissue able to perceive pain? Nature is certainly not haphazard. Pain, at least acute pain, serves as a warning system. Pain is a sense or nerve function that warns the body of immediate danger that threatens the body's integrity. The body must take action and avoid this danger or harmful situation. From this perspective, pain certainly is useful; in some cases it is life saving.

The International Association for the Study of Pain (IASP) defines pain as "an unpleasant sensory and emotional experience associated with actual or potential tissue damage, or described in terms of such damage". In this definition, the warning function of pain is clearly identified.

The word "pain" originates from Greek word "poena", which means a fine or penalty. In Greek mythology, pain is used by the Gods to punish misbehaving mankind.

Acute versus chronic pain

Acute pain usually signifies an intensive here-and-now pain. Its cause in most cases easily can be identified. Chronic pain is more difficult to define. The term chronic signifies a longstanding condition; by "longstanding" some researchers mean 2-6 months. Today, many researchers working with pain realize that pain may be chronic from the outset. This means that the time factor is overridden by other factors as etiology, symptomatology, and response to treatment. Other researchers state

11

Acute Pain	Chronic Pain
1. Often has a cause (inflammation in 85%)	1. Cause is difficult or impossible to define
2. Starts suddenly	2. Starts insidiously and slowly
3. Pathology can be found	3. Pathology rarely can be found
4. Patient is anxious and afraid	4. Patient is bitter and depressed
5. Easy to treat	5. Difficult or impossible to treat
6. Good response to analgesics	6. Poor response to analgesics

Fig. 1. The differences between acute and chronic pain.

that chronic pain has nothing to do with the pain *per se* and that other terminology should be used. Chronic pain, they argue, is a mental disease akin to depression.

The differences between acute pain and chronic pain are outlined in Fig. 1.

Although differences outlined in Fig. 1 simplify the distinction somewhat, they do suggest some of the factors that distinguish acute pain from chronic pain.

Classification of pain

In dentistry, many different types of pain are described because many structures and types of tissue are involved. Dental pain can be classified as follows:

Duration
- acute
- subacute
- chronic

Site of pain generation
- central pain (from central nervous system)
- visceral pain (from organs)
- peripheral pain

Pain distribution

- local pain (site of origin)
- referred pain (felt in another region than where generated)
- projected pain (felt in normal area of innervation but generated somewhere along the nerve fiber or nerve root

Pain localization

- toothache
- headache
- facial pain
- back pain, etc.

Pain type

- inflammatory pain
- rheumatic pain
- muscular pain
- vascular pain
- neuralgic pain
- cancer pain

References

1. Merskey H, Bond MR, Bonica JJ et al. Classification of chronic pain syndromes and definition of pain terms. Pain Suppl 1986; 3: 1-222

CHAPTER 1

Basic principles of pain physiology

Peripheral nociception

The term nociception originates from Greek word "nox", meaning harm or damage. By nociception is meant all processes that originate in the periphery and lead to pain sensation. The peripheral pain receptor, which most often is a thin, unmyelinated (naked) nerve fiber, is thus termed the nociceptor. All of the tissues in the body except the brain and the enamel of the teeth contain nociceptors.

The pain process can be described the following way (Fig. 2).

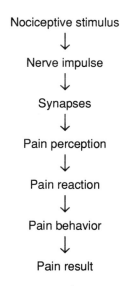

Nociceptive stimulus
↓
Nerve impulse
↓
Synapses
↓
Pain perception
↓
Pain reaction
↓
Pain behavior
↓
Pain result

Fig. 2. The normal pain process.

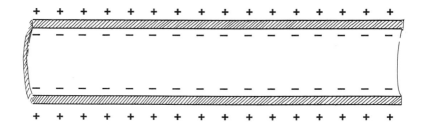

Fig. 3. The resting polarized nerve cell.

A resting nervecell is *polarized*, i.e., there is a positive charge on the outside of the cell membrane and negative charge on the inside of the cell membrane (Fig. 3). This is due to active processes in the cell membrane (e.g., sodium pump) and a difference in ion permeability.

When a stimulus acts upon the nerve cell, Na^+ rush into the cell through special, now-opened sodium ion channels due to high concentration of Na^+ on the outside of the cell. This brings a positive charge to the inside of the nerve cell, and a depolarization that causes an electric current to travel along the nerve cell membrane. This process is called the nerve impulse or action potential. The nerve cell will repolarize immediately after the action potential has passed by an outward diffusion of

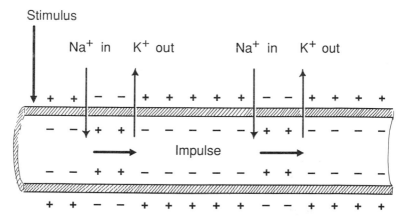

Fig. 4. Depolarization and repolarization of the nerve cell.

Table 1

Nociceptive stimuli capable of acting upon a nociceptor

- inflammation
- infection
- trauma (stretch, compression, crush)
- chemicals (acids, alkalines)
- biochemical mediators (histamin, bradykinin, prostaglandins, H^+, K^+, serotonin, norepinephrine, etc.)
- thermal factors (cold, heat)
- actinic factor (ultraviolet or infrared rays)

---

many K^+. Later on, the surplus of the Na^+ will be pumped out of the cell again, against a concentration gradient while K^+ at the same time slip into the cell in order to maintain the osmotic equilibrium. This process requires energy - the energy that is converted into the electric impulse (Fig. 4).

Different types of stimuli can act upon the nerve cell membrane (Table 1).

Inflammation is nature's response to every local stimulus or irritant. It is the first element of the healing process that works to repair tissue damage by the stimulus. The five *cardinal* symptoms of inflammation are:

- *tumor* = swelling (due to edema)
- *rubor* = redness (due to vasodilation)
- *calor* = warmness (due to filling of blood)
- *functio laesa* = decreased function, i.e., trismus
- *dolor* = pain (due to release of chemical mediators)

Although inflammation is useful insofar as it is the first step of the healing process, the symptoms of inflammation are unpleasant to the patient. One could say that treatment of acute pain is the same as antiinflammatory action.

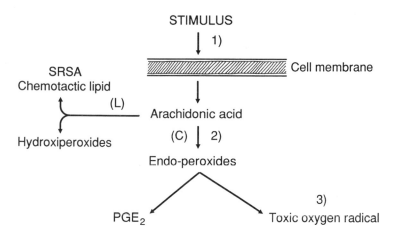

Fig. 5. The prostaglandin synthesis.

Some of the most intriguing biochemical mediators in inflammation and pain are the *prostaglandins*. They are formed from cell walls stimulated in inflammatory processes (Fig. 5).

The end products, especially the PGE_2, cause pain. The PGE_2 lowers the threshold of the nociceptors to other stimuli. The free oxygen radical O, which actually is a free oxygen atom, is inflammatory and tissue damaging in nature; it will seek another free oxygen radical in order to form an oxygen molecule. The analgesic effect of paracetamol (acetaminophen) and to a certain degree of diflunisal is thought to be due to a neutralization of the toxic oxygen radical. The analgesic effect of acetylsalicylic acid (ASA) and other nonsteroidal antiinflammatory drugs (NSAIDs) are due to inhibition of the enzyme *cyclo-oxygenase* (C), which catalyzes the prostaglandin synthesis. In effect, all the peripheral-acting analgesics (ASA, paracetamol, NSAIDs, phenazone, etc.) act by inhibiting the formation of prostaglandins. The cell membrane can be stabilized by either glucocorticosteroids or local analgetics (that is how they establish analgesia). If a cell membrane is treated with either drug, before it is stimulated or irritated, it is stabilized and will act

17

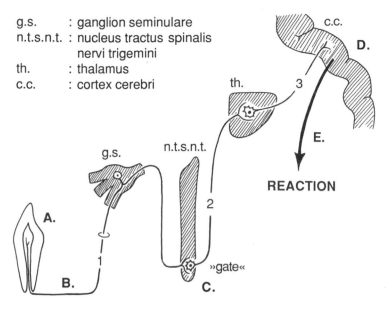

g.s. : ganglion seminulare
n.t.s.n.t. : nucleus tractus spinalis nervi trigemini
th. : thalamus
c.c. : cortex cerebri

Fig. 6. The classic pain tract from a tooth to the cerebral cortex, involving three neurons.

accordingly: Fewer or no prostaglandins are formed, so the patient experiences less pain and less swelling after an operation.

This knowledge is bacic to understanding *pain prophylaxis* and *edema prophylaxis.*

Pain tracts

The classic pain tract consists of three neurons connected in the synapses (Fig. 6). The electric pain message is in the synapsis transformed to a chemical message as a chemical transmitter substance is released from the presynaptic neuron, crosses the synaptic cleft, and affects the postsynaptic neuron, where the pain transmission continues or is perceived (Fig. 7).

The electric pain impulse is transformed into a chemical message in the synapses and back into an electric action potential in the postsynaptic neuron. The release of the chemical pain transmitter substance P can be blocked

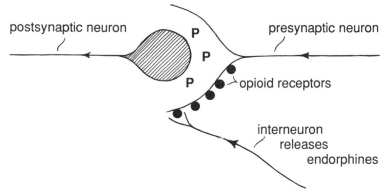

Fig. 7. Chemical pain transmitter substance, P.

by naturally occurring morphine-like substances called endogenous morphines, or *endorphins*. When endorphins are released from small interneurons close to the presynaptic neuron, they attach to opioid receptors on the presynaptic neuron and block the release of substance P, thus blocking further pain transmission. If this important pain-controlling system malfunctions, chronic pain can result. Some instances of chronic pain related to depression have been shown to be characterized by lower-than-normal concentrations of endorphins in the spinal fluid. The interneurons are especially found in the substantia gelatinosa in the dorsal horn of the medulla spinalis and in the brain stem.

These interneurons probably can be activated by both *peripheral means* and *central means*.

The peripheral control is activated when mechanoreceptors are stimulated, e.g., by needle acupuncture or by electrical stimulation, or TENS (transcutaneous electrical nerve stimulation).

The central control is activated from some cells in the area around the aquaductus cerebri (PAG = periaquaductal gray substance). This area, in turn, is activated from the cortex cerebri, from the hypothalamus, and from reflex loops from the ascending pain tracts. Also, exogenous administered opioids (morphine, meperidine) can activate the PAG cells and thus the descending central

19

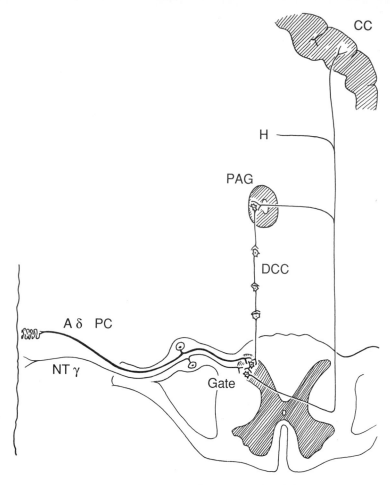

Fig. 8. Schematic drawing of the principle of the "gate control theory", where the gate is situated in the dorsal horn of the spinal medulla.

Explanation of abbreviations:

Aδ: A-delta fibres stimulated by touch, vibration, acupuncture, or high frequency TENS

NTγ: Non-specific pain-transmitting gamma-fiber

PC: Peripheral control

DCC: Descending central control

PAG: Peri-aquaductal gray substance

H: Connections with higher centers in midbrain and brain stem

CC: Cerebral cortex

pain control. The convergence of both the peripheral and the central control in the back horn is called the "gate" (see Fig. 8).

If a pain tract is activated many times, pain tract "printing" probably can take place. That is, the pain tract is easily remembered by the nervous system. Next time something happens in the periphery close to the nociceptors of the printed tract, it is likely that the specific tract is activated, and the patient experiences pain to stimulus that otherwise would be subliminal. Pain tract printing is believed to be one source of chronic pain arising in the periphery after acute pain, and also to be involved in postoperative pain. General anesthesia blocks pain perception in cortex cerebri by removing the consciousness. The pain tract, however, is intact during surgery. The brain remembers the pain tract after the anesthesia wears off, and the patient experiences postoperative pain and discomfort in the area. Blocking the area of surgery with analgesics apparently prevents the pain tract printing. In experiments using analgesics for this purpose, patients without exception, have experienced less postoperative pain and swelling.

Pain perceptions

Pain perception is pain experience, which happens in the cerebral cortex. The perception of pain is a process that remains unexplained; we do know that the participation of consciousness is necessary. If consciousness is removed by general anesthesia, the brain will still perceive pain by the usual pain mechanisms but the mind will be unaware of it. This perception can be registered by monitoring blood pressure and pulse during general anesthesia. Whenever painful procedures are performed, blood pressure and pulse frequently rise, and it becomes necessary for the anesthesiologist to administer more general anesthetic in order to keep the patient quiet and motionless. It is, therefore, wise to block the pain tract peripherally, by administering local analgesia in the field of surgery, in order to minimize the central input of painful impulses. Blocking the pain tract will decrease the risk of postoperative pain and edema and ensure a more even and smooth general anesthesia.

Pain perception can be measured objectively using sophisticated computer EEG (electroencephalography), whereby small spikes (EVP = evoked potentials) are identified and correlated to pain stimulation. It is still too early to evaluate the clinical significance of this finding, but the process - the first objective measure of pain perception in the brain - is certainly interesting.

The area of the cerebral cortex (gyrus postcentralis) devoted to facial and masticatory pain occupies about 25% of the total area of the brain handling pain perception. This fact illustrates the significance of facial pain and demonstrates the priority the brain gives this region. This fact also must help explain why oral pain is so common.

Pain reaction

Pain reaction is the body's reaction to pain perception. Pain reaction is usually both

- *physiological* and
- *psychological.*

Physiological pain reaction is autonomic response and includes rise in blood pressure and pulse, sweating, paleness, nausea, vomiting and motor withdrawal (pain reflex).

Psychological pain reaction includes the crying, fear, or anger that may accompany pain perception.

Pain reaction varies widely from person to person, and also will vary within the same person depending on that person's will of mind and body, and time of the day. Some generalizations also can be made about variations in pain perception based on sex and race. Since pain is an individual, highly personal response, it is important for the dentist to treat every pain report as valid. Recall that tissue damage is not necessary for patient pain.

Pain reaction can be lessened by sedatives, nitrous oxide, alcohol, morphine, hypnosis, and suggestive relaxation measures, and increased by fear, depression, previous bad experiences, and unpleasant behavior of dental team members.

Pain threshold

Pain threshold is an imaginary factor. It is defined as being inversely proportional to pain reaction, i.e., the more pain reaction the less pain threshold and vice versa. When talking about the pain threshold it is important to define the parameters.

The pain *perception* threshold is the least stimulus that will elicit a painful sensation. This parameter usually can be defined precisely in an individual, is not dependent on previous administration of acetylsalicylic acid, but will increase if morphine is given.

The pain *tolerance* threshold is defined as the stimulus value that is unbearable to the patient, i.e., the point at which the patient will not tolerate more pain. This value is dependent on both acetylsalicylic acid and morphine and other analgesics.

In daily practice, the dentist is interested in raising the pain threshold in order to make it possible for the patient to undergo painful treatment.

References

1. Bell WE. Orofacial pains: Classification, diagnosis and management. Chicago: Yearbook Medical Publishers Inc, 1985.
2. Bond MR. Pain Its nature, analysis and treatment. Edinburgh: Churchill Livingstone, 1979.
3. Melzack R, Wall PD. Pain mechanisms: A new theory. Science 1965; 150: 971-9.
4. Snyder S. Drugs and neurotransmitter receptors in the brain. Science 1984; 224: 22-31.

CHAPTER 2

Basic principles of pain psychology

Dental patients would best be served by dentists adopting the following working definition of dental treatment pain:

> An unpleasant sensory and emotional experience associated with actual or potential tissue damage, or described in terms of such damage

Pain is a highly subjective experience. Dentists often are faced with trying to ameliorate pain that is inconsistent with the pathology observed. *Treating Fearful Dental Patients* describes, for example, a patient who found the pain of a coronal polish with a rubber cup "unbearable". It is important to keep clear the two-step task of the dentist: first, the patient's pain must be acknowledged and accepted; and second, the pain must be treated. As clinicians our observation is that we often deny the validity of the patient's report and thus fail to manage the pain well. Research demonstrates, for example, that patients receive too little pain medication. From the patient's perspective, all pain reports are very real. This central fact we cannot change. What we can do is use a broad spectrum of psychological and pharmacological techniques to control pain. To restate, as clinicians we need a large repertoire of skills to manage pain. Throughout this text, references will be made to matching this set of skills to the individual patient's problems.

Central and peripheral components of pain

It is remarkably simple, as a clinician, to begin to act as if pain control consists only of blocking neural transmission in peripheral nerves. After all, most of our effort goes into the technique of local analgesia. However seductive this approach, it ignores much of what is known about pain. It is quite clear that pain has both peripheral and central (brain and brain stem) components.

Role of patient background

Much famous work on cultural background and pain has dealt with this peripheral-central interaction. There are classic studies, for example, showing Jews, Italians, and Scandinavians as having similar pain thresholds, the initial level where peripheral nerves will fire. However, these ethnic groups were found to have quite different pain tolerance reactions. Their behavior during the pain experience varied depending on their upbringing. Clinically speaking, many patients will endure pain - say drilling without local analgesia - because that is what is expected of them; others, in the same situation, will refuse treatment. Both groups feel pain but react to the noxious stimulus differently. Since a clinician cannot change a patient's background, a clinician must be sensitive enough to adapt technique to a particular patient. Stereotypic treatment is not helpful to the individual.

Prior experience

We know that prior experience is an important factor in predicting how effective local analgesia will be. Previous difficulty getting numb has a strong predictive relationship to failures in analgesia at future dental visits. *Drug-sophisticated* addicts and those who abuse alcohol are also difficult to get numb. Again, prior experience - a form of drug tolerance - may be at play. Similar evidence suggests that patients develop tolerance to nitrous oxide analgesia, for some this analgesia will decrease in effectiveness over time.

Placebo

Clinicians should regard the placebo as an additional clinical tool that makes use of suggestion in managing pain. Research has shown that about 35% of surgical patients receive adequate pain relief with placebo alone and that placebo pain agents are about 54 to 56% as effective as morphine. The effectiveness of the placebo effect is directly proportional to the analgesic to which it is being compared. Higher dosages work better than lower dosages; injections are more effective. However, patients with chronic anxiety may not respond well to placebos.

Setting

We also are aware today of the important effect the dental setting has on pain perception. Patients will report more pain and tolerate the same pain worse at the dental clinic than at home or in research lab. In much the same way, soldiers wounded in battle are less likely to request pain-control drugs than patients in the hospital, even though the soldiers' wounds are far worse. For the soldier, the wound is the mark of hero and a ticket home. For a patient, the pain only means disability and time lost from work and family responsibilities. Once again, we cannot charge this response to noxious stimuli but we can accept and understand it. This understanding will keep us from withholding pain-control medications when often they are needed.

References

1. Milgrom P, Weinstein P, Kleinknecht R, Getz T. Treating Fearful Dental Patients. A Patient Management Handbook. Reston: Reston Publishing Co., 1985.
2. Turk DC, Meichenbaum D, Genest M. Pain and behavioral medicine. A cognitive behavioral perspective. New York: The Guilford Press, 1983.

CHAPTER 3

Pain relief principles

Every patient who suffers from pain desires relief from that pain. The patient expects the dentist to remove the pain, whatever its nature. When this is not possible, patients are disappointed and occasionally even become aggressive. Pain relief can be looked upon as *pain treatment* and *pain prevention.*

Pain treatment

Pain treatment, the most common form of pain relief, is relieving already-existing pain. The abbreviation *p.n.* stands for pro necessitate, or "taken as necessary". If a patient suffers from pain constantly or over a long period of time, it is important that the plasma level of a chosen analgesic at all times be kept above the minimum therapeutic level, so the patient is kept pain free. If the drug concentration is allowed to decrease below the minimum therapeutic level, the patient starts to feel pain. To increase the threshold again to pre-pain level, it normally will take a *higher* dose than the dose that would have maintained the plasma concentration above the therapeutic level. It is therefore important for the dentist to know the half-life and bioavailability of the drug used, so the right dosage and administration interval can be determined. In this way, the maximum benefit of the drug with the minimum dosage is obtained (Fig. 9).

Pain prevention

Pain prevention or pain prophylaxis is a new principle aimed at preventing anticipated pain from "breaking through". The principle is based on the finding that it is

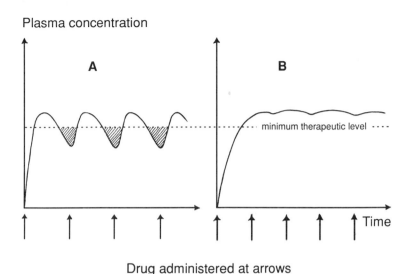

Plasma concentration

A

B

minimum therapeutic level

Time

Drug administered at arrows

Fig. 9. (A) Insufficient pain control with a drug with short half-life. The marked areas below the minimum therapeutic level signify pain. (B) Sufficient pain control with a drug with long half-life. The same effect could be obtained with the drug in (**A**) by shortening the interval of drug administration.

easier to keep a patient pain free than to remove existing pain.

If in oral surgery, a patient is administered a systemic analgesic, i.e., paracetamol or an NSAID, before the local analgetic is given, the plasma concentration of the systemic analgesic will be sufficient to prevent the pain from breaking through postoperatively. The pain threshold is kept at a higher level and, if the systemic analgesic is acting peripherally at the site of pain origin, pain tract printing will be prevented. Pain prevention can be aided by blocking an area of surgery after the actual procedure has ended with a long-acting local analgetic, such as bupivacaine or etidocaine. Local analgesia will stabilize the cell membranes and decrease production of prostaglandins as well as decrease the so-called axon-reflex, which originates in the area of surgery and ends at

29

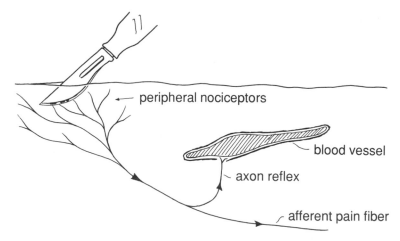

Fig. 10. Vasodilation caused by stimulation of peripheral nociceptors.

the blood vessels in the same area causing vasodilation and thus edema and more pain (Fig. 10). In short, surgical pain creates more pain and edema, and it is important to stop the pain where it originates. Local analgesia should always be used together with general anesthesia in order to cut pain tract printing at the peripheral level. Pain prophylaxis is more effective and less drug consuming than traditional p.n. pain treatment.

Information to the patient

Probably the single most important factor in controlling pain is informing the patient. He or she should know:

- what the likely diagnosis is
- whether there is more than one diagnosis
- the recommended treatments and any alternatives, including no treatment
- the possible treatment consequences and risks
- the prognosis and benefits of treatment
- the cost of the procedure

The information should be easily understood by the patient. If the patient is afraid, the explanation should *not* involve sensitive or emotional words (e.g., blood, cut, chisel, suture); the dentist should try to find words that have the same meaning but not the potentially frightening connotations (e.g., liquid instead of blood, open instead of cut, divide instead of chiseling, close instead of suture). Explanations may be illustrated with drawing or pictures.

Note in your records what you have told the patient. Remember, your records are legal documents.

It is essential that the patient understands what you say. As far as pain treatment is concerned, never promise the patient that he or she will not experience pain; say instead that you will do your best to leave the patient pain free. In fact, patients will have less anxiety if you promise to work as hard as you can on effective pain control.

Cold pressor test

Before exploring the issue of patients' pain, you might find it useful to learn something about your own response to pain. Place your hand in a bucket full of ice and water. Keep it there for five minutes.

How did you handle the pain you experienced?

What did you think about?

Could you keep your hand in the bucket?

References

1. Chapman PJ. Postoperative pain control for outpatient oral surgery. Int J Oral Maxfac Surg 1987; 16: 319-24.
2. Hill CM, Carroll MJ, Giles AD, Pickvance N. Ibuprofen given pre- and postoperatively for relief of pain. Int J Oral Maxfac Surg 1987; 16: 420-24.
3. Rosenquist JB, Nystrom E. Long-acting analgesic or long-acting anesthetic in controlling immediate postoperative pain after lower third molar surgery. Anest prog 1987; 34: 6-9.

CHAPTER 4

Psychological methods of pain relief

The key psychological factor in controlling pain is accommodating patient preference. Patients develop preferences for any number of reasons, such as past experience and cultural and personality factors. It is important to have available several different approaches to meet these various needs.

A dentist may employ a strictly pharmacologic solution to operative pain control using local analgesia. At the other pole is the use of a purely psychological technique such as hypnosis. Strategies may be combined, such as using distraction and local analgesia. Of course, no technique is purely pharmacologic or psychological. Even the patient who depends on local analgesia is cognitively or psychologically active. What is different about patients who employ psychological strategies is that they plan to use strategies they have practiced beforehand. Even the patient who employs only psychological means for controlling pain in fact has the help of natural opiates in the brain that centrally mediate pain perception. What we are really doing in selecting pain-control strategies is helping patients find what works for them.

Often practitioners adopt styles of pain control that they attempt to use with all patients. Note for example the difference between Northern European and North American practitioners. The former use relatively little local analgesia for operative dentistry while the latter employ it almost universally. This is not particularly effective patient care since it ignores individual differences. Undoubtedly, an examination of each case would reveal that some of the Northern European patients who did not receive local analgesia were obviously uncomfort-

33

able. By the same token, many of the North American patients probably could have tolerated brief periods of drilling without analgesia - and might have preferred it that way.

Choosing a pain-control strategy begins with ascertaining patient preferences: What have been the patient's past experiences? Has pain control been adequate? What strategy does the patient use in life to manage pain? Does he or she take a pain killer for a headache or lie down and rest? Does the patient use both a pharmacologic, e.g. aspirin, and a psychological approach, e.g. .rest? Asking such questions will reveal how the patient approaches pain.

What pain-control strategies, the practitioner should learn, does the patient already have available? Some patients can readily identify strategies they already know. Women may be familiar with the breathing techniques used in natural childbirth. Patients may use stress-reduction strategies like Transcendental Meditation, yoga, or self-hypnosis. Children and adolescents can readily distract themselves.

The dentist should explain to patients that they must be active while being treated, even if peripheral or centrally active pain-control drugs are used. Explain the link between the brain and felt physiological reactions: We see a sad movie and cry; we see a motor vehicle accident and feel nauseous. The pain experience has similar components. Because of this link, it is important that patients have psychological strategies to employ.

Some patients refuse to learn psychological strategies - wishing only local analgesia - and to remain passive. This approach is fine,as long as the patient feels comfortable - little movement, normal pulse and respiration. Similarly patients may employ only psychological means for pain control as long as they are comfortable and allow the dentist to proceed.

Remember that pain is a major factor in dental fear. This fear keeps patients from being regular users of care and from obtaining the oral health benefits of modern preventive dental care. The choices the practitioner makes about pain control are very important.

Evidence indicates that the particular technique adopted by a patient is not important. Rather, the patient must believe its efficacy and have practiced it beforehand. Some patients also find it helpful to have a second, backup technique available in case their primary strategy is not working.

Distraction

The most basic and helpful techniques available to dentists and patients are distraction techniques. Many strategies, such as the use of music, video, taped stories for children, and white sound, are primarily distraction techniques. The fundamental clinical principles behind distraction are:

- patients should choose what distraction they think will work for them
- distraction alone will work best on pain of lower intensity and shorter duration
- the more involving the distraction is, the better it will work
- patients should have control over the distraction. For example, if music is used, the patient should control the volume.

Working with adolescents and older children
Most children can daydream. To distract some children it is only necessary to ask them to think of a favorite TV program or to *play* a video in their head. Others can readily imagine a game or sport. Encourage the child's involvement by asking for details. Ask about the video or the sport. The clinican should not be passive!

Working with adults
Music and other taped material often works well. An in-

office system is helpful as a backup for patients without strong preferences. However, it's better for the patient to choose the distractor. For example, have the patient go to a music store and purchase a tape he or she always has wanted to hear. Have the patient bring the unopened tape to the dental appointment and listen to it for the first time there. The office will need to have portable tape player and earphones available. More elaborate in-office video systems or electronic games also are helpful for some patients.

One patient that surprised us was a woman who could not tolerate the pain of a polishing cup on her teeth. She bought a tape of Mark Twain stories about dentistry at an audio store. Listening to this tape she was able to tolerate care.

Relaxation and breathing

The dentist should explain to the patient that physically relaxed patients tolerate pain better than those who are tense. In fact, much research has shown that responses even to pulp testers are different in clinic and nonclinic settings. The two exercises below are most adaptable to the dental setting. Patients need to practice these exercises at the clinic and at home in order to have them work maximally at a dental appointment.

Progressive relaxation can be used just before the dentist begins and during difficult times in an appointment. Have the patient practice tensing and releasing individual muscle groups for 5 - 10 seconds each. Some clinicians prefer to focus only on the upper body - hands and arms, shoulders, neck, jaw, facial muscles - and others relax the whole body beginning at the feet. Most important, the patient should learn the difference between tense and relaxed. The dentist or assistant who teaches these strategies should practice them along with the patient (Fig. 11).

At a real appointment the patient should be allowed in the operatory a few minutes early and asked to practice

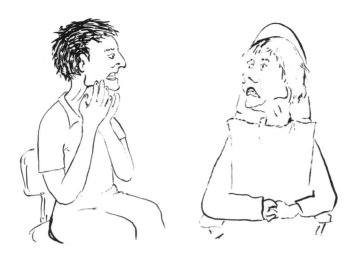

Fig. 11.

the relaxation skill. If the clinician notes the patient tensing during treatment, he or she should stop for a moment and encourage the patient to practice the exercise.

Practicing relaxation techniques with the patient is much more effective than simply urging the patient to practice!

Paced, slow breathing is both very relaxing and very distracting. In a slow, quiet voice, the practitioner should instruct the patient to take a very deep breath, hold it for 5 seconds, and exhale slowly over a count of 5 seconds. Coach the breathing by keeping a hand on the patient's shoulder and gently depressing the hand during exhalation.

Most patients tense and hold their breath during painful procedures such as injections. Slow breathing is an antidote, for particularly tense situations, have the patient imagine breathing like waves.

The goal of this strategy, of course, is physical relaxation. The exact pattern of breathing is unimportant. Patients can be encouraged to focus their efforts on techniques that will work.

Timing

Timing also affects the patient's experience of pain. When performing potentially painful procedures such as injections or bursts of drilling, begin when the patient is most relaxed, e.g., on the exhalation cycle.

The practitioner should explain to the patient how long the procedure will last. It is better to tell a patient the procedure will last 5 minutes and stick to that time than to say "it will be only a little longer". If the procedure is technically demanding and takes longer than planned, take a short rest break before proceeding. Structuring the appointment that way is a very effective pain-control adjunct. Break up the time spent on the procedure into small bits. For example, doing 5 two-second bursts of drilling is better than doing a single 10-second burst.

Hypnosis

Hypnosis is an extension of the breathing relaxation and distraction approaches outlined above. It combines these strategies with suggestions, given by the clinician, for comfort, warmth, pain control, amnesia, and other sensations. It works best when patients believe in it and it works better when they practice.

A form of hypnosis called guided imagery is very useful in the clinic. Ask the patient to pick a scene somewhere pleasant, such as a particular beach or forest trail. With each set of breaths, suggest that the patient think of details of the scene, such as the clouds in the sky, noises of the water, smells, etc. Give the suggestions in a calm, slow voice. Doing this is also relaxing for the clinician. This technique works well in conjunction with paced breathing and other relaxation techniques (Fig. 12).

Proceed with dentistry only after the patient is calm. If the patient is having difficulty coping, a short break and reinstruction usually will suffice.

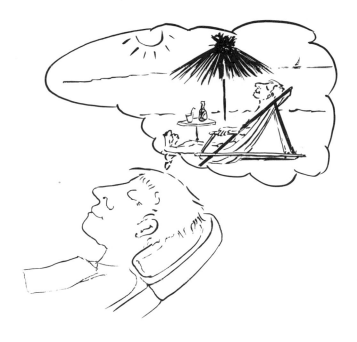

Fig. 12.

Other more complicated hypnotic-induction strategies are available for those who are interested.

Drug tolerance

One important justification for using psychological, rather than pharmacologic, approaches to pain control concerns the phenomenon of tolerance. Studies have shown that many pain-control agents become less effective with individual patients over time. The reasons behind this phenomenon are not known. However, we do know that relying strictly on drugs can be a risky clinical strategy. This is particularly true with patients who may drink alcohol heavily or abuse drugs.

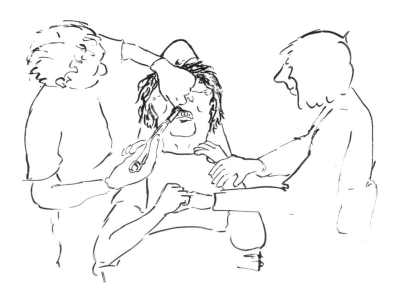

Fig. 13.

Desensitization

This *in vivo* procedure can be helpful for patients who are afraid of injections of a local analgetic. Begin by teaching them the relaxation and breathing skills discussed earlier. Then construct a hierarchy of steps leading to an injection - such as putting on topical analgetic, seeing the syringe, holding the syringe, having the syringe in place with the plastic cap on the needle, etc. (Fig. 13).

Rehearse each step, from least to most fearful, while the patient practices breathing and relaxation. Do not proceed to the next step until the earlier one is mastered without any upset. Use this procedure in a separate appointment from one in which you intend to provide dentistry to minimize the pressure on the patient.

Stress inoculation

This psychological technique involves presenting the patient with several ways to cope with pain - relaxation, distraction, breathing, etc. - and allowing them to practice each technique. The practice might involve the patient's experiencing the pain of placing a hand in an ice bucket or simply inflating a blood pressure cuff on the patient's arm. In theory, the patient can use this approach to deal with treatment pain. This technique is not readily adaptable to dental clinical practice without considerable preparation.

References

1. McCaul KD, Malott JM. Distraction and coping with pain. Psych Bull 1984; 95(3): 516-33.
2. Milgrom P. Behavioral methods and research issues in the management of the adult dental patient. Anesth Prog 1986; 33(1): 5-9.

CHAPTER 5

Basic pharmacologic approaches

Premedication

There are two basic purposes of premedication in outpatient dental practice: postoperative pain control and anxiety reduction. There is often confusion about the choice of agents resulting from lack of clear purpose of the therapeutics.

Postoperative pain control

Ample clinical evidence indicates that a preoperative dose of an analgesic, especially a nonsteroid antiinflammatory drug is helpful in reducing or controlling postoperative pain after oral surgery, endodontics, and periodontal surgery. The usual dose is ibuprofen (200-400 mg), or acetaminophen (650 mg). The rationale for the premedication is that peak blood levels are achieved 1 to 2 hours after oral administration. Thus, administration 1 hour before a procedure is likely to result in more postoperative comfort.

There is little evidence that narcotic analgesics have any advantage over the nonsteroidal drugs, and they cause more side effects. Further there is little evidence that antibiotics prevent any pain associated with dental surgery. There is also no indication for the use of barbiturates or benzodiazepines for pain control.

Reducing anxiety

To a large extent, fear and anxiety cause pain and discomfort through psychophysiological mechanisms (such

Table 2

Premedicant drugs for anxiety

Drug	Usual dose 1 hr before bed
Flurazepam	15-30 mg
Lorazepam	2-4 mg
Triazolam	0.25-0.50 mg
Nitrazepam	5-10 mg

All doses should be reduced 50% in the elderly

as headache and tension) or predispose the anxious patient to feeling pain. Most anxious patients will do better if they practice a physical mechanism to achieve relaxation. However, for some individuals, typically those who present with *generalized anxiety,* drug adjuncts are appropriate. Such patients have multiple sources of stress in their lives and perceive themselves as nervous. They will frequently report sleeplessness, nausea, or similar psychophysiologically based symptoms.

Malamed recommends using a benzodiazepine before bed as the appropriate adjunctive drug. The choice of drug should be based on a lack of active metabolites (reducing the hangover effect), fairly rapid onset, and a sedative hypnotic effect. According to Malamed, four drugs most clearly meet the needs of dentists: Flurazepam, lorazepam, triazolam, and nitrazepam (or temazepam, a similar drug) (Table 2).

In our clinical experience, triazolam has the greatest potential among these drugs. Its peak plasma levels are achieved in just over 1 hour and its half-life is only 2.2 hours. Patients fall asleep in about 30 minutes. It produces little residual drowsiness. Triazolam may be administered orally or sublingually.

In contrast, lorazepam has a half-life of 15 hours; flurazepam and nitrazepam have half-lives of almost two days. Temazepam, has a very slow onset, making it of questionable value in the clinic. Benzodiazepines potentiate the adverse effects of alcohol and other drugs, so care must be taken in prescribing. Allergy also is a problem for some patients.

Considering how effective oral benzodiazepines are in producing sleep, there is little rationale for giving other agents such as barbiturates, which not only are less effective clinically but also carry many more risks. Benzodiazepines are not available in rectal suppository form in some countries. They are available in injectable form for IM administration, but there seems little reason to use this approach.

Local analgesia

Local analgesic agents, when used effectively, facilitate the delivery of high-speed, efficient, and comfortable dental treatment. The injection of the analgetic is seductively easy, and the presumption that the drug will block peripheral nerve conduction and thus pain, is made all too easily. There is, however, growing evidence that failure to achieve optimal analgesia is a common clinical problem.

In a survey of general dentists, 90% recalled at least one analgesic failure during restorative dentistry during the past week, and the failure rate averaged 13.1% of all restorative visits. Visits were prolonged because of patients complaining about pain and from 2 to 10% of patients in individual practices had to have treatment terminated earlier than planned without completing the work. The failure rate varied by area: 88% of dentists had at least one failed mandibular block; maxillary posterior (42%); maxillary anterior (26.2%); mental (9.5%); and intraligamentary (10.7%). For a parallel study, a random sample of patients in the community were asked how effective local analgesia was. Not surprisingly, 13.7% reported not being "numb" during drilling. Many patients reported they had previous difficulty with analgesia and/or were afraid of injections. The correspondence between clinician and patient data suggests the validity of this clinical problem.

Thus, the focus of this chapter will be on five subjects: when to use local analgetics and which ones to use, moderating the pain of injection, areas to be anesthetized, injection devices, and dealing with analgesic failure. There are many fine textbooks on local analgesia pharmacology and technique, which this brief chapter cannot replace.

When to use local analgetics

Restorative dentistry

Adequate analgesia for cutting dentin requires careful attention to drug choice. At least 60-90 minutes of pulpal analgesia is appropriate. Drug formulations that produce this are lidocaine 2% with 1:80,000 or 1:100,000 epinephrine; lidocaine 4% with 1:100,000 epinephrine; mepivacaine 2% with levonordefrin, and prilocaine 4% with 1:200,000 epinephrine. For especially lengthy appointments such as for fixed prosthodontics, bupivacaine or etidocaine should be considered (discussed below under oral surgery and tooth impactions). Mepivacaine 3% or prilocaine 4% are shorter acting and may be used for cementation.

Periodontics

For treatment involving only soft tissue and root planing, pulpal analgesia is less important. Drug formulations to be considered here are mepivacaine 3% and prilocaine 4%. When osseous surgery is contemplated, lidocaine 2% with 1:50,000 epinephrine provides good control of hemorrhage at the injection site. Note, however, that the 1:50,000 formulation may be a less effective anesthetic than the 1:80,000 or 1:100,000 epinephrine drug. This formulation also can be given using an intraligamentary syringe for papillary injection. Surface agents may be

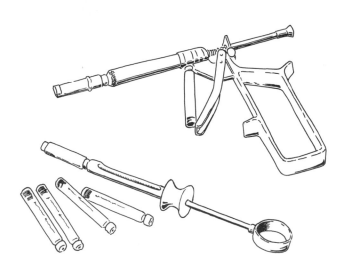

Fig.14.

useful for many patients for scaling or for dressing changes or suture removal.

Endodontics

Lidocaine 2% with 1:100,000 epinephrine or its equivalent (see restorative drugs) is appropriate. In endodontic pain control, a larger field should be anesthetized then with other procedures. Intrapulpal injections are likely to be more effective using the drug with 1:50,000 epinephrine and using an intraligamentary syringe (Fig. 14). For off-hour emergencies, bupivacaine 0.5% with 1:200,000 epinephrine will provide up to 12 hours of pain control and reduce the need for peripheral or central-acting analgesics.

Oral surgery and impactions

Surgery for routine extractions does not appear to require particularly profound analgesia even though many patients appear to react to the elevation of a tooth.

Appropriate drug formulations may be similar to those in periodontics: mepivacaine 3% or prilocaine 4%. These drugs may be helpful for an incision, drainage, and surgical impactions. Surface agents may also be helpful in this situation or for removing sutures.

It has been argued that longer-acting analgetics are useful here for two reasons. First, they are effective agents for longer procedures; and second, they allow time for peripheral pain-control agents to take effect before numbness wears off. The most available drug for dental use in this category is bupivacaine 0.5 % with 1:200,000 epinephrine. There is little evidence, however, that this strategy reduces the need for postoperative analgesics.

Moderating the pain of injection

Injections are the most feared aspect of dental care; paradoxically, most of the anxiety dental patients experience is associated with pain of injection.

To achieve a comfortable injection, the patient must be prepared and relaxed. The dentist should not hide the syringe, as this raises the suspense and worry a patient experiences, which may, in turn, increase pain. Often a patient will hold his breath during an injection, so it is helpful to coach the patient in paced breathing (see Chapter 4 on psychological methods of pain control).

Topical analgesia should always be used, and the patient should be told why it is being used. Putting some on the patient's tongue, and letting the patient poke himself with a cotton swab, can be helpful to demonstrate its effect.

Most often surface analgesia is achieved using a topical paste. Typical pastes contain 5% lidocaine and 2% amethocaine, 5% lidocaine and 0.015% hyaluronidase, 10 -20% ethyl aminobenzoate (benzocaine) or 2% tetracaine. All of these agents are effective if left on dry tissue at least two minutes. Most clinicians do not wait long enough for the drug to work.

Analgesic solutions containing 0.5 - 2% amethocaine HCL, 0.5 -2% cinchocaine HCL, 5 - 10% cocaine HCL, or 4% lidocaine HCL can also be used as long as care is taken to contain them.

Analgetic squirt or spray bottles that dispense 10 mg per squirt can be helpful in procedures such as suture removal. Extreme care must be used to avoid overdose.

Many of these drug formulations taste terrible. Try to taste any new topical drug and avoid using it, if possible, if its taste is bad.

Jet injectors

These devices provide controlled amounts (0.2 - 0.4 ml) of analgetic by pressure to areas 5 mm to 1 cm in diameter. Using them does not appear to cause pain although their action may scare some patients. Care should be taken to avoid moving the device and traumatizing tissue.

Ethylchloride

The use of refrigerant sprays is relatively ineffective, painful and potentially dangerous to the patient. Since duration of analgesia is very short, it may provide adequate pain control for injection. The fumes of refrigerant sprays are dangerous, and the chilling may be uncomfortable to surrounding teeth. Such sprays are not recommended.

Factors associated with pain of injection

Every dentist should aim for painless injections. Much pain is caused by carelessness: the major source of pain is the sudden distension of tissue caused by too-rapid injection of large volumes. Rates of 1 ml per 30 seconds are desirable in sensitive areas, such as the upper anterior.

Explain the concept to patients using the analogy of a water pistol: squirting the pistol hard and fast at one's hand is painful; squirting out a dribble is not. Informing patients in this way will lessen their anxiety about injections.

Clinical mythology abounds regarding needle gauge and temperature of solutions. Evidence suggests 25- to 30-gauge needles are no different. Room-temperature and body-temperature solutions are no different clinically. Solutions from the refrigerator should be warmed.

In locations such as the hard palate, apply pressure before injection to cause blanching of the tissue. This pressure provides a substantial degree of surface analgesia. The pressure can be applied with a cotton swab or mirror handle. With multiple-palatal injections, only the first block injection should be in unanesthetized tissue; the others should be at the border of previously numb area, with the dentist extending analgesia in stages until the desired result is achieved.

Areas to be anesthetized

It is our belief that many problems are iatrogenic/dentist caused. One way to minimize some of these problems is to anesthetize an area somewhat larger than the minimum needed.

Upper arch

For single teeth, either a supraperiosteal infiltration or periodontal ligament injection (PDL) is appropriate. For multiple teeth, many PDL injections are time consuming. Rather, a posterior superior alveolar block and/or posterior, middle, or anterior superior alveolar infiltrations should be used. Nasopalatine nerve or greater palatine nerve blocks should be used for optimal analgesia on the palatal tissue. The routine use of block injections is likely to be more efficient and provide superior analgesia than infiltrations alone. Analgesia of palatal tissue is especially

49

important in both restorative dentistry and periodontics. Our experience is that many dentists avoid these injections because they are unplesant to give. This results in unnecessary patient pain.

Lower arch

PDL injections have been moderately successful for single teeth. Supraperiosteal infiltrations are rarely satisfactory. For multiple teeth, an inferior alveolar block must be supplemented with lingual and buccal blocks. The Gow-Gates and Akinosi approaches offer the advantage of achieving a mylohyoid block. These may need to be supplemented with a buccal block. The PDL injection is a useful supplement to all injection procedures.

Injection devices

For conventional analgesia, an aspirating syringe with 25-30 gauge disposable needle is used. Periodontal ligament injections may be given with conventional syringes, but the special-purpose PDL syringes offer many advantages (Fig. 14). The special devices allow solutions to be injected under considerable pressure and have closed or protected barrels in case of cartridge breakage. The PDL syringe accepts regular cartridges; lidocaine 2% with 1:50,000 epinephrine using a 30-gauge needle is most effective. If a conventional syringe is used with high pressure, first wrap the cartridge with autoclave tape.

All injection devices should be autoclaved before use and stored in a sterile container. Needles should be disposable. Solutions should be checked for expiration date and discarded if old, discolored, or damaged in any way.

Dealing with analgesia failure

Preventing failures is essential to successful analgesia practice. Keys to success include:

1. Choose an agent that provides the appropriate length of analgesia for the procedure. Don't make patients wait for long periods, or pulpal analgesia may decrease.
2. Use the appropriate amount of analgetic solution. As much as 1.8 ml of 2% lidocaine, 1:100,000 epinephrine may be needed for an infiltration and 3.6-5.4 ml for a mandibular block. Sometimes more solution is needed.
3. Cover an adequate area; do not leave tissues in the working field unanesthetized.
4. Don't waste time; onset of most local analgetics is 90 to 180 seconds. If analgesia symptoms are not beginning, especially in the mandible, evaluate the need for additional injections or an alternative injection technique.
5. Recall that pulpal analgesia time is very short for some techniques such as the PDL, (approximately six minutes). Supplementary injections may be needed if restorative procedures are being carried out.

Recall that pain is a personal, subjective perception of the patient. Thus, if attempts to achieve analgesia are not successful, operative procedures should be postponed and the analgesia approach reevaluated. Patients with a history of analgesic failure should be identified before treatment. Special attention should be directed to patients with a history of illicit drug use or alcohol abuse who may be particularly difficult to anesthetize. A special testing appointment, during which you demonstrate your ability to control pain, may be helpful. In this case select an easy tooth, anesthetize it fully and carefully, and perform various tests - hot, cold, pulp tester, etc. - to ascertain pain control. Be sure to rule out fear as a source of responses. Do not carry out any operative procedure at this appointment. Rather, use the appointment to gain patient confidence in your techniques. Proceed with care the next visit. With such patients, all procedures with analgesia must be administered with great care.

References

1. Allen GD. Dental anesthesia and analgesia (local and general). 3rd ed. Baltimore: Williams and Wilkins, 1984.
2. Bennett CR. Monheim's local anesthesia and pain control in dental practice. 7th ed. St. Louis: The CV Mosby Co., 1984.
3. Malamed SF. Handbook of local anesthesia. St. Louis: CV Mosby Co., 1980.
4. Malamed SF. Sedation - a guide to patient management. St. Louis: CV Mosby Co., 1985, Chapter 8.
5. Roberts DH, Sowray JH. Local analgesia in dentistry. 2nd ed. Bristol: John Wright and Sons Ltd., 1979.

CHAPTER 6

Nitrous oxide analgesia

Understanding nitrous oxide

Nitrous oxide (N_2O) affects the brain in two ways:

- analgesia
- sedation

The two effects are different and should not be confused. As an analgesic, nitrous oxide is quite effective: 30% N_2O in equilibrium after about 6-8 minutes of administration offers an analgesic activity that equals the administration of 10-15 mg of morphine s.c. Note, however, that the key word is "equilibrium", i.e., the tissues are saturated with nitrous oxide, so alveolar uptake and release are identical. If a painful procedure is started too early, the analgesic effect will certainly be unsatisfactory. The analgesic effect of N_2O is thought to be the result of stimulation of the presynaptic opioid receptors, since the analgesic effect can be reversed by the narcotic antidote, naloxone, that blocks these receptors.

The sedative effect of nitrous oxide is less well understood but is believed by many to be due to a stabilization of certain neuron cell membranes in the brain stem and cortical areas involved in consciousness. The sedative effect mimics the action of diazepam, which is believed to have a GABA (Gamma-amino-butyric-acid) receptor backgound. GABA is a general central-nervous-system inhibitor. The sedative effect of N_2O occurs rather quickly, i.e., in a couple of minutes, which may cause the practitioner to believe that the treatment can begin. Although nitrous oxide can provide heavy sedation, it cannot alone induce general anesthesia. Nitrous oxide should always be used with oxygen, and the concentration of oxygen in the inhaled mixture should never be allowed to be less than 20%, which means that the concentration of nitrous oxide never can surpass 80%. Actually, the optimum effect, with the least side effects, is reached at about 50% N_2O after equilibrium.

If a patient is stimulated before the effect of the nitrous oxide is sufficient, the patient will sometimes overreact to the stimulus. This is called a "paradoxical excitation", since the reaction is unexpected. This reaction is probably provoked by selective depression of inhibiting neurons, which results in the exciting neurons dominating the response to the stimulus. This phenomenon can occur with all CNS-depressive drugs administered in insufficient dosages. Only when the dosage is correct will *all* the neurons be depressed and the patient satisfactorily sedated.

Indications and contraindications

Nitrous oxide can be used with advantage to:

- provide analgesia in painful procedure
- provide relaxation and sedation to the slightly nervous patient
- provide, in combination with other drugs (barbiturates, narcotics, halothane), general anesthesia.

There are very few *absolute* contraindications to nitrous oxide, one, of course, being nasal obstruction due to a cold or hay fever. Another absolute contraindication is first-trimester pregnancy; a risk, however slight, of miscarriage has been pointed out in some studies.

There are some *relative* contraindications. Nitrous oxide may not be ideal for patients who:

- are undergoing psychiatric treatment
- are unable to cooperate
- are very old and very young
- have a family history of malignant hyperthermia
- are very upset or anxious

Administration

Certain rules should be followed for the safe and effective administration of nitrous oxide.

1. Start the procedure with inhalation of 100% oxygen 6 liters per minutes (preoxygenation phase). This increases the safety by causing higher oxygen tension in the tissues and increases the efficacy, since the nitrous oxide will diffuse more quickly from the alveolar atmosphere into the blood.
   During this period, coach the patient in effective breathing. The technique suggested earlier for paced breathing and relaxation is appropriate. Most anxious patients would benefit from a practice session using the gas before the actual appointment where it is to be used clinically.
2. The key to good nitrous oxide analgesia is *slow* induction. The concentration of N_2O should be increased slowly; "Crash induction" should be avoided. The following routine demonstrates slow induction.
   Inhalation of a total gas flow per minute from 6-8 liters, mixed as:

   1 liter N_2O + 5 liters O_2 for 1 minute
   2 liters N_2O + 4 liters O_2 for 2 minutes
   3 liters N_2O + 3 liters O_2 for 3 minutes

3. The maintance-phase mix should consist of 50% N_2O and 50% O_2 in total gas flow of 5-7 liters per minute, depending on the patient size.
   Note: Advise the patient that he can control the gas concentration by mouth breathing. Always watch the patient's respiration and skin color. If the patient reacts violently to the nitrous oxide or feels he is losing control, turn the gas off immediately.
4. A few minutes before the treatment is over, turn the nitrous oxide off and allow the patient to breathe pure oxygen (6-8 litres per minute) for 3-4 minutes

(postoxygenation phase). This will eliminate the risk of diffusion hypoxia, a condition that results from a patient breathing normal atmospheric air that contains only 21% O_2, since the alveoli in the lungs quickly fill with the N_2O streaming out of the blood.

Safety

If the above-mentioned rules are followed and the anesthetic equipment is in order, no acute or life-threatening situation is likely to arise.

Most countries today require the equipment for outpatient care to adhere to the following specifications:

- administration of O_2 must never decrease below 20%; in the United States, 50%
- if the oxygen pressure drops during use, the flow of nitrous oxide is automatically turned off (fail safe) and the patient is allowed to breathe room air
- a reservoir bag of at least 1.5 liter should always be attached
- the gas machine should be equipped with a scavenger device removing exhaled air from the patient, so the dental staff is not exposed to high concentrations of nitrous oxide over a prolonged period.

With regard to the safety of the dentist and the clinical assistant, it is safe to work with nitrous oxide, if:

- the scavenger device is efficient
- the patient does not exhale through the mouth
- the room's air ventilation is good (air renewal 3 times per hour).

Studies have shown that if these rules are not adhered to, an increased risk of miscarriage or decreased male fertility may result.

56

References

1. Cohen EN, et al. Occupational disease in dentistry and chronic exposure to trace anesthetic gases. J Amer Dent Assoc 1980; 101: 21-31.
2. Langa, H. Relative analgesia in dental practice. Philadelphia: WB Saunders, 1976.
3. Malamed SF. Sedation -. A guide to patient management. St. Louis: CV Mosby Co., 1985.
4. Yang JC, Clark WC. Antagonism of nitrous oxide analgesia by naloxone in man. Anaesthesiol 1980; 52: 414-17.

CHAPTER 7

General anesthesia

Conscious sedation

General anesthetics allow the dentist to treat the anxious patient undergoing a traumatic procedure. The rationale for using these agents is rarely pain control per se; rather, it is the combination of an aversive procedure and patient need. The use of general anesthetic agents lessens, but does not eliminate, the need for active patient participation in the dental procedure. The less the patient is able or willing to cope, the greater the role of the pharmacologic agent. Similarly, the longer and more aversive procedure often decreases the patient's ability to cope effectively.

The development of local analgesia and sedative drugs such as the benzodiazepines now offers an alternative to general anesthesia. Anxiety and pain can be relieved while the patient remains conscious.

This text is aimed at general practitioners who are not likely to work in a setting where these drugs will be needed and thus are not apt to acquire the specialized skills required for their use. Nevertheless, a fundamental understanding of these agents is important if the generalist is to advise his or her patients and refer to specialists. For those who use these agents, this brief review will provide an update on both efficacy and safety.

The use of these new pharmacologic techniques to relieve patient anxiety is common in oral surgery practice. The techniques involved the use of single agents and various combinations of agents.

Use of conscious sedation has several goals: The patient must remain conscious with relief of anxiety and pain. Protective reflexes must remain intact with only small changes in a patient's vital signs. Amnesia for the procedure may make a patient less anxious about the subsequent treatment and has been considered desirable.

The drugs currently used for sedation not only produce desirable clinical effects but also may cause effects such as cardiovascular and respiratory depression or prolonged recovery.

Efficacy and safety of intravenous benzodiazepine sedation

Benzodiazepines have been used effectively to sedate patients. These agents enhance the effect of gamma-amino-butyric-acid (GABA), which is a central nervous system inhibitory transmitter.

Intravenous diazepam has been used because it produces rapid onset of sedation with minimal cardiorespiratory effects. The major disadvantages of using diazepam for outpatients are its long half-life, pharmacologically active metabolites, and significant incidence of thrombophlebitis at the injection site. A relatively new benzodiazepine, midazolam, offers several advantages over diazepam. Midazolam is a water-soluble benzodiazepine that has a rapid onset, 1-2 minutes, and a short elimination half-life of 2-5 hours. Patients who receive midazolam are adequately sedated and suffer less thrombophlebitis and more complete amnesia than would occur with diazepam.

When used clinically, intravenous benzodiazepines are titrated to the desired level of sedation. Administration is slow (1 mg/ 30 sec - 1 min). The desired effect is slurred speech and half ptosis (droopy eyelids). The average sedative dose is 10-12 mg for diazepam and 2.5-7.5 mg for midazolam. Evidence suggests that IV drugs of this type can potentiate lidocaine toxicity.

Efficacy and safety of intravenous benzodiazepine and narcotic sedation

Narcotic analgesics are sometimes administered with sedatives to decrease a patient's perception of pain. Although narcotics are effective analgesics, they cause cardiac and respiratory depression. Meperidine (pethidine) or fentanyl most commonly are used. Fentanyl has a short half-life, 30-40 minutes, and causes less histamine release than does meperidine.

Narcotic agonist-antagonists, such as pentazocine, nalbuphine, and butorphanol, are now also used because they cause less respiratory depression than meperidine. The narcotics also have been combined with benzodiazepines to potentiate their action and decrease the total dose of drug needed to sedate a patient. However, the efficacy of combining narcotics with these drugs has been questioned.

A typical dose of meperidine is 37.5-50 mg. An average dose of fentanyl is 0.05-0.06 mg. Depending upon body-weight, a typical dose of butorphanol is 1-2 mg; of nalbuphine 7-8 mg; and of pentazocine 20 mg. The narcotic drugs usually are given before the benzodiazepine, which is titrated after 2-4 minutes. Doses of benzodiazepine are halved when used in conjunction with narcotics.

Efficacy and safety of ultra short-acting barbiturates

Small incremental doses of barbiturates such as methohexital commonly are used for sedation. The barbiturates suppress the central nervous system by inhibiting the reticular activating system. Ultra short-acting barbiturates have a rapid onset of action and rapid recovery. However, it can induce general anesthesia and is a cardiac and respiratory depressant. Patients given benzodiazepines with narcotics experience significantly more respiratory depression than when given benzodiazepine alone.

Methohexital is given in 5-10 mg amounts to desired sedative effect. Duration is 5-7 minutes before redistribution. When given with other drugs methohexital is administered last. The combination of barbiturate and narcotic drug is the most dangerous combination.

When using these drugs, the dentist must take a careful medical history and be cognizant of contraindications. These drugs should not be used by untrained individuals. In many parts of the world, special licensing requirements govern use of these drugs.

References

1. Beirne OR. Current and future research in dental sedation and anesthesia. Anesth Prog 1986; 33: 193-96.
2. Bennett CR. Conscious sedation: An alternative to general anesthesia. J Dent Res 1984; 63: 832-33.
3. Dionne RA. Differential pharmacology of drugs used for intravenous premedication. J Dent Res 1984; 63: 842-47.
4. Dionne RA. Methodological needs and pharmacologic research with adult dental patients. Anest Prog 1986; 33: 50-54.
5. Dixon RA, Kenyon C, et al. Midazolam in conservative dentistry. Anesth 1986; 41: 276-81.
6. Korttila K. Clinical effectiveness and untoward effects of new agents and techniques used in intravenous sedation. J Dent Res 1984; 63: 848-52.
7. Malamed, SF. Sedation. A guide to patient management. St. Louis: CV Mosby 1985; pp 342-48.
8. Malamed, SF. Conscious sedation and general anesthesia techniques and drugs used in dentistry. Anesth Prog 1986; 33: 176-78.

CHAPTER 8

Analgesics

Analgesics are administered to relieve pain, most commonly after the pain has started. Rather than this, a "curative" approach, it might be preferable to take the analgesic before the expected pain occurs, e.g., preoperatively. Analgesics taken prophylactically will suppress the pain, even before it begins, and also act as an antiinflammatory agent to decrease swelling and edema. Consequently, the patient likely will have a higher pain threshold, and total analgesic consumption probably will be lower.

The key to modern pain control with analgesics is that pain prevention is better than pain treatment.

Analgesics are classified into two categories, depending on site of action, peripheral acting and central acting.

The peripheral acting analgesics inhibit the synthesis of prostaglandins (Fig. 5). The central acting analgesics activate presynaptic opioid receptors, thus blocking the release of substance P in pain transmission (Fig. 7). Morphine is also known to exert action on some cells in the periaquaductal gray substance (PAG), which is the center for descending fibers that end in the dorsal horn, in the "gate", and are able to shut off the pain transmission at this level (Fig. 8).

Table 3 offers an overview of the analgesics.

Centrally acting analgesics

Buprenorphine

Buprenorphine is synthetic morphine and is more potent than natural morphine. One advantage is that it can be administered sublingually in small "resoriblets" that dissolve and allow the active principle to be absorbed

Table 3
Analgesics

A. Centrally acting analgesics

Strong/Addictive:	Weak/Slightly addictive:
buprenorphine	dextropropoxyphene
morphine	codeine
pethidine (meperidine)	
ketobemidone	
pentazocine	

B. Peripherally acting analgesics

Antiinflammatory/ GI irritation:	Little or no antiinflammatory action/GI irritation:
salicylates	paracetamol (acetaminophene)
NSAIDs	phenacetine
diflunisal	

C. Neuroleptic

levomepromazine

through the thin oral mucous membrane into the richly vascularized submucosa. It is well suited for patients with severe acute pain, but should not be given to patients with little pain, as it is likely to cause vomiting. Dosage is 0.2 mg resoriblets 3 to 4 times daily for severe pain.

Morphine

Morphine is without doubt the most important and potent of the central-acting analgesics. Despite many new synthetic and semisynthetic opiates, morphine is still the one of choice for treating severe pain. Morphine is best administered subcutaneously (SC) or intramuscularly (IM), but in hospitals it is often given intravenously (IV).

For strong cancer pain, morphine can be given perorally in larger dosages to compensate for the "first passage" effect in the liver. Since the liver breaks down much of the drug before it reaches the main circulation the oral dosage must be increased 60-80% over the parenteral dosage. Morphine is administered in dosages of 10-15 mg SC or IM. It often is used in combination with diazepam and scopolamine to premedicate patients before surgery.

Pethidine (meperidine)

Pethidine is a synthetic narcotic, well absorbed by all routes. It mimics morphine in all respects, although its action probably is shorter. Pethidine is most often given parentally in dosages of 50-100 mg.

Ketobemidone

The primary advantage of this drug is easy peroral administration in dosages of 25-50 mg.

Pentazocine

The original goal in developing this drug was to create a narcotic with the benefits of morphine but without the side effects and misuse potential. Thus far, the attempt has not succeeded. Pentazocine has the same side effects as morphine, and in addition can cause euphoria and hallucinations. It has both analgesic and antagonist properties and can be administered orally; the usual dosage is 50-100 mg.

Dextropropoxyphene

Dextropropoxyphene has been quite popular for some time, either used alone, or in combination with acetylsalicylic acid (ASA), phenacetin, or other compounds. The sustained release form of this drug is often used by older people with chronic arthritic pain. Recently, several factors have diminished its popularity. It is being misused by drug-addicted persons when they cannot obtain narcotics. It has strong cardiotoxic action in combination with ethylalcohol and is responsible for many suicides. Finally, its analgesic action on acute pain can be disputed. It is probably fair to state that dextropropoxyphene is not indicated in dental practice today.

Codeine

Codeine is the most widely used oral analgesic, usually in combination with ASA or paracetamol. The analgesic dosage is 50-100 mg. Codeine is 3-methylmorphine and is demethylated to morphine in the liver. For each 10 mg codeine, 1 mg of morphine is formed, reputedly the basis of its analgesic action. Codeine has a lower abuse potential than most other narcotics; overdose will induce nausea and vomiting.

Peripherally acting analgesics

Salicylates

The best know salicylate is undoubtedly acetylsalicylic acid (ASA, aspirin). ASA has very good analgesic actions, as it is a powerful inhibitor of prostaglandin synthesis. It also has antipyretic, antigout, antiinflammatory, and antirheumatic actions. Unfortunately, ASA has quite a few side effects such as GI irritation, with the risk of ulcer formation and occult bleeding into the GI tract. ASA can cause allergic type reactions such as Reyes syndrome. It should never be given to children. The dentist should know that ASA interferes with normal coagulation, and can cause abnormal bleeding patterns following surgery. ASA, therefore, is contraindicated at the time of oral surgery. The optimal dosage is 0.5-1 g; the maximum adult dosage is 5 g a day. ASA often is combined with codeine, a logical combination as ASA acts peripherally and codeine centrally to produce a synergistic action.

NSAIDs

NSAIDs stands for nonsteroidal antiinflammatory drugs, perhaps better known as the antirheumatic agents. They are quite popular and often used in dentistry. NSAIDs can be given postoperatively without any risk of causing bleeding, and also can be used for pain prophylaxis. The only side effect seems to be GI irritation. Naproxen and ibuprofen are two of the most popular NSAIDs, but there is probably little difference in action and side effects among the drugs in this class.

Diflunisal

Diflunisal is an NSAID, but is mentioned separately due to its long half-life. Twice daily administration in 500-mg dosages is sufficient, and lessens the risk of patient non-compliance. It can be used during surgery, although it has some slight antithrombotic action.

Paracetamol (acetaminophen)

This popular drug also is known as acetaminophen. It has reasonably good analgesic effects and few side effects, if the *optimum dosage is not surpassed*. Paracetamol is the natural breakdown product of phenacetin and has fair analgesic effect in dosages of 0.5 to 1 g. Maximum daily adult intake should not exceed 6 g. Overdosage (12 g or more) can damage the liver irreparably, especially in combination with alcohol. Paracetamol has no action on coagulation and can therefore be used to treat postoperative pain and discomfort. It is often combined with codeine, and even can be given to infants.

Phenacetin

Phenacetin is the "P" in an APC-combination, where A stands for ASA and C for caffeine. Recently, its use has been disputed, as many think it might cause damage to the kidneys when taken over a long period. This question has not been resolved, but until further notice it is wise to reduce phenacetin intake and substitute it with paracetamol in correct dosage.

Glucocorticosteroids

Commonly called steroids, these drugs are characterized by pronounced antiinflammatory action, inhibiting both edema and pain. Their action is supposed to stabilize the cell membrane towards the inflammatory stimulus, inhibiting the release of prostaglandins. Blood vessels are stabilized also. The most popular steroid is dexamethasone, which can be injected sublingually into the oral tissues in a dosage of 4 mg just before surgery.

Levomepromazine

This drug is a neuroleptic with sedative and analgesic actions. Because of its strong sedative effect, it should only be used for nighttime analgesia. It can be combined with narcotics with some advantages. Its analgesic action is probably due to pain dissociation, i.e., the patient can feel the pain but does not care about it.

References

1. Parkhouse J, Pleuvry B, Rees JMH. Analgesic drugs. Oxford: Blackwell Scientific Publications, 1979.
2. Seymour RA, Walton JG. Pain control after third molar surgery. Int J Oral Surg 1984; 13: 457-85.
3. Troullos ES, Freemann RD, Dionne RA. The scientific basis for analgesic use in dentistry. Anesth Prog 1986; 33: 123-38.

CHAPTER 9

Stimulation-produced analgesia

The term stimulation-produced analgesia (SPA) means analgesia caused by some kind of stimulation, or in the words of Melzack and Wall, "closing the gate for pain transmission". Most people instinctively use SPA, for example after hitting the fingers with a hammer, a person is likely to shake and rub the hand vigorously, and perhaps to blow on it. These stimuli activate mechanoreceptors in the skin, muscles, joints, and periosteum in the damaged area, and the impulses travel centrally in thicker nerves (A-beta fibers) than do the pain impulses (A-delta and C-fibers). When they enter the dorsal horn of the spinal medulla or the trigeminal nucleus in the brain, small interneurons lying close to the presynaptic pain transmitting neurons release endorphins that subsequently block the pain transmission by blocking the presynaptic release of substance P (Fig. 15).

Acupuncture

Special sensitive points of the body can be stimulated with small needles. Careful rotation or vibration of the needles can induce a sensation of warmth and analgesia after 10-20 minutes of stimulation. Healers in India originally described this principle, which was adopted and refined by the Chinese *many* thousand years ago. A modern adaptation called electro-acupuncture applies electrodes to the needles and uses currents to stimulate the sensitive points.

When acupuncture was introduced to the West in the beginning of the 1970's many scientists and clinicians looked upon this principle with wonder and skepticism.

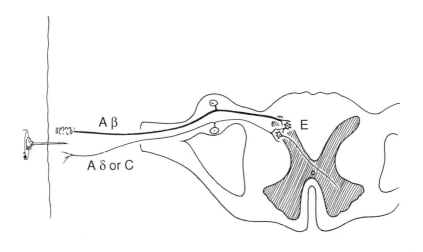

Fig. 15. The gate control mechanism.

Not anymore! Acupuncture is now used all over the western world, and is being seriously investigated in many institutions and research centers.

Acupuncture cannot solve all pain problems for all patients. Certainly, there is a wide variation of response to acupuncture analgesia, depending on the skillfulness of the acupuncturist and the patient's ability to obtain a positive placebo effect. As a general rule, acupuncture always can be attempted to evaluate its efficacy. It is normally harmless; the only risk would be penetration of the lungs in the upper thoracic regions, if the needles are inserted too deeply. In some patients, the response is long-lasting following just one treatment. In other patients the analgesia is very short, lasting perhaps one hour, and perhaps requiring many treatments.

·Generally speaking, the earlier acupuncture is started, the greater the efficacy. The ancient Chinese claimed that acupuncture could be used prophylactically against various diseases.

Many of the acupuncture points of the body correspond to myofascial trigger points, that is the points or areas of referred pain from deeper lying muscles, tendons, or joints. It is not possible to demonstrate these points anatomically. They should thus be considered physiologic points with a special concentrated ability to perceive stimuli. Interestingly enough, many acupuncture points in the face coincide with points of referral of pain from teeth with chronic closed pulpitis.

In dental practice, acupuncture might be indicated in patients with myofascial pain syndrome, atypical trigeminal neuralgia, herpes zoster, and other ill-defined chronic pain conditions. Acupuncture has been used as an analgesic during painful dental treatment with varying degrees of success.

Transcutaneous nerve stimulation

The analgesic action of TNS or TENS is based upon the same principle as acupuncture. However, needles are not used; instead electrodes are placed on the skin over the painful area and a current is passed through the region between the electrodes. TENS should never be administered to patients with pacemakers! At least two different types of TENS exist.

Conventional high-frequency TENS

An AC current with a frequency of 50-200 Hz and an intensity of 20-30 mA usually will provide almost immediate but rather short-lasting (1-2 hours) analgesia. There is no effect on the muscles due to the high frequency rate. Naloxone (a morphine antagonist), administered to the patient after analgesia is obtained, has no effect on the analgesia. Like acupuncture, high-frequency TENS probably exerts its analgesic action by closing the gate.

Low-frequency TENS

An AC current with a frequency rate of 2-4 Hz is applied, producing muscle contraction. Analgesia can be obtained after 15-20 minutes of stimulation and can last up to 24 hours. Naloxone will immediately revert the analgesia to pain, indicating that the endorphin system is involved. High concentrations of spinal endorphins measured after low-frequency TENS give support to this theory.

If TENS is administered preoperatively, e.g., before surgical removal of impacted lower third molars, both an analgesic and antiedematous effect can be shown. If the TENS treatment is continued postoperatively, the need for other analgesics decreases or disapperars. Other indications for TENS include toothache, sinusitis, and muscle pain. Nitrous oxide is a helpful adjunctive treatment.

References

1. Gersh MR, Wolf SL. Applications of transcutaneous electrical nerve stimulation in the management of patients with pain. State-of-the-art update. Physical Ther 1985, 65. 314-35 (very extensive literature list).
2. Katch EM. Applications of transcutanously electrical nerve stimulation in dentistry. Anest Prog 1986; 33: 156-60.
3. List T, Helkimo M. Acupuncture in the treatment of patients with chronic facial pain and mandibular dysfunction. Swed Dent J 1987; 11: 83-92.

CHAPTER 10

Physical methods of pain control

Pain can be controlled with certain physical methods that usually are simple and easy to administer. As a general rule, physical methods should never be overused.

Heat

Heat dilates the blood vessels and increases circulation in an area of inflammation. This principle is of importance in all cases where pain has led to tissue ischemia. Decreased circulation will result in accumulation of metabolic products, especially lactic acid, which lowers pH and causes pain and sustained spastic muscle contraction. Application of heat can break this vicious circle.

Heat can be applied by using simple hot packs, infrared lamps, and ultrasound. Surface application of hot packs will not produce deep penetration of the heat, but will give a feeling of comfort and relaxation in the area. Heat treatment sessions should never exceed 15 minutes. Too much heat can worsen the symptoms.

Cold

Application of cold is advantageous in the acute phase of traumatic and surgical pain. Many believe the action is caused by vessel contraction, which is probbably not true as the tissue temperature 5 mm beneath a cold ice pack is normal. The application of cold causes arteriole contraction in the superficial layers, but a slight dilation in deepest layers due to compensatory mechanisms. The analgesic action of cold probably is due to two factors. In the superficial layers the lower temperature will decrease nerve function, but the principal action is most likely caused by an activation of temperature receptors resulting in a closure of the spinal gate. Similar to the mechanism of acupuncture. The self-perpetuating pain circle sustained by the axon reflex (pain causes vasodilation that again causes edema and more pain) is thus broken by the application of cold, which might explain its anti-edematous effect.

Cold can be applied with an *ice pack over* the painful site, but should only be used for the first 24 hours after pain has started. In dental practice, *ethyl chloride* administered in a spray bottle can be applied as it evaporates at a temperature of 12°C. Football and athletic coaches also use it to treat players who sprain a muscle or tendon. Ethyl chloride should not be used intraorally.

Controlled destruction of pathological tissue is accomplished by using cryosurgical equipment to apply extremely low temperatures. Temperatures of -80°C can be reached using nitrous oxide. Cryosurgery has had success in treating otherwise intractable typical trigeminal neuralgia, where either the infraorbital or mental nerve is destroyed by the extreme cold at the respective exit points of the nerves. Interestingly, the normal nerve function without pain seems to reappear after 3-6 months. The nerve might regenerate as the low temperatures do not destroy the nerve sheath (the Schwann's sheath).

Laser therapy

Laser therapy, particularly the soft laser, has gained increasing popularity in recent years. The principle is that the concentrated light energy (laser = *l*ight *a*mplification by *s*timulated *e*mission of *r*adiation) will activate molecular movements in the cells and thus increase local heat and speed up metabolic processes. Soft laser may give relief in cases of acute traumatic and surgical pain. There is no risk to soft laser, except that eye damage can occur if a person looks directly into the laser beam.

73

Physiotherapy

Physiotherapy is an important treatment for muscular and temporomandibular joint (TMJ) problems. Physiotherapy can be applied passively as massage of tender muscles, and more actively as jaw exercises. In case of muscular developed trismus or constriction of the opening movement, the PNF method can be attempted (PNF = proprioceptive neuromuscular facilitation). The patient tries to open the jaw against resistance applied with the hand beneath the base of the mandible. Following strong activation of jaw opening muscles (the lateral pterygoid, the supra- and infrahyoid, and the digastric muscles), the jaw closing muscles (the masseter, medial pterygoid, and temporal muscles) will relax due to reflexes from the mesencephalic nucleus of the trigeminal nerve. As the trismus is caused by spastic contraction of the jaw closing muscles, the reflex will break this spasm and allow normal function to return.

In case of severe clicking from the TMJ, the patient should be taught to restrict the opening movements to pure rotation or hinge movement. The patient should avoid the anterior sliding movement of the condyles over the articular tuberculum. TMJ problems and myofascial pain conditions can in most cases be relieved symptomatically by bite splints, but it is important to remember that such therapy rarely is curative, and should be followed by a careful analysis of the jaw function and occlusion.

References

1. Bell WE. Orofacial pains: Classification, diagnosis and management. 3rd ed. Chicago: Year Book Medical Publishers, 1985.
2. Ramfjord SP, Ash MM. Occlusion. Philadelphia: WB Saunders Company, 1966.
3. Zarb GA, Carlsson GE. Temporomandibular joint. Function and dysfunction. Copenhagen: Munksgaard, 1979.

CHAPTER 11

Special dental pain conditions

Acute pulpitis

This section has three parts: examination; emergency pain control; and treatment of pulpitis.

Examination

In most cases it is not difficult to identify the tooth causing the pain. The purpose of the exam is to confirm that the origin of the problem is the pulp, as treatment may be different if the origin is periodontal abscess or cracked tooth. The exam should consist of a periapical radiograph, visual-tactile inspection, periodontal probing, percussion, hot/cold and electric tests. The tooth with primarily a pulpal problem will not have the characteristic narrow and deep periodontal pocket of a tooth fracture. The root fracture may mimic most other signs of pulpal involvement. Root fractures are largely attributed to guttapercha condensation, although pin and post placement, impact injuries, and intracoronal cast restoration placement also are implicated. Thus, fractures may be largely ruled out by history.

Biting forces are implicated in crown/root fractures in posterior teeth. Often these teeth are vital, and pain may be elicited by having the patient bite on a Burlew wheel. Pain occurs on biting and is relieved when the pressure is released. The limited crown fracture is likely to respond to placement of an orthodontic band. More severe fractures should respond to the same emergency treatment as described in the following paragraphs.

Emergency pain management

The goal here should be to reduce the discomfort of the pulpitis, control infection and allow the patient some rest and nutrition. We have observed that many dentists are too eager to open teeth in the acute situation, causing more discomfort. Moreover, alternative strategies permit the staff to plan the procedure and allow enough time in the schedule. The clinical rationale for this approach also stems from evidence that treatment of teeth with pre-operative pain is likely to increase the probability of postoperative pain.

If the tooth has an open carious lesion, use of 10-20% benzocaine gel is an effective topical pain control agent. If there is no open lesion, the tooth may respond to a field block with a long-acting local analgetic such as bupivacaine or etidocaine. Pain medication should be dispensed immediately. Nonsteroidal antiinflammatory medications such as ibuprofen (400-600 mg), aspirin (1000-1200 mg) or diflunisal (500 mg) are effective. Acetaminophen (paracetamol, 1000 mg) is a less effective agent because of a longer delay in activity but may be acceptable if local analgesia is used. Caution should be exercised in using narcotic drugs because of the side effects. There is some evidence that 10 mg codeine combined with ibuprofen, aspirin, or acetaminophen may be marginally better than narcotics for pain.

Opioids, such as codeine phosphate, pentazocine, dextropropoxyphene, and morphine alone are uneffective pain control agents in dentistry. Dihydrocodeine causes "hyperalgesia", nausea, and drowsiness. Zomepirac sodium (50 mg) is an effective agent but has been taken off the market in the US because of adverse effects. Caution should be exercised in using this drug.

A medication to promote sleep (such as triazolam 0.25-0.50 mg) may be prescribed. Its onset is rapid, so the patient must have an escort or wait to take the medication after arriving home.

If there is evidence of a periapical swelling or the patient is febrile, antibiotics may be prescribed. The trend is toward larger initial doses (penicillin V, 2 g stat and 500 mg every 6 hours orally). Alternative medications are erythromycin, cephalosporins, or metronidazole. A drug allergy history should be taken. These antibiotics are taken up more efficiently on an empty stomach. Note, however, that erythromycin may cause significant nausea. If nausea is a problem, prochloroperazine (25 mg) suppositories or tablets may be used. Such drugs have the added benefit of promoting sleep. Warm rinses will often provide symptomatic relief. Caution patients not to place hot packs on the face or to use products such as aspirin topically.

Treatment of pulpitis

The consensus of endodontic specialists is that the complete instrumentation and debridement is the ideal emergency treatment of involved teeth. For this reason it is important to quiet immediate acute pain so that time can be set aside for proper treatment. In addition, local analgetics are likely to be more effective in the well-rested patient. The outcome of partial pulp treatment is unpredictable.

Extraordinary means should be used to gain effective local analgesia, for example, blocks and supraperiosteal (infiltration) injections, which may be supplemented with intraligamentary injections. Injections should be given very slowly (1 ml/min). The pulp tester may be an imperfect aid to gaining solid pain control. Topical analgesia should be used.

The tooth should be opened with a new, very large bur, using short bursts of 1-2 seconds rather than continuous drilling. Allow the patient short rest breaks (15-30 seconds) between bursts. Tell the patient that the bursts will be short so he or she does not anticipate longer discomfort. Intrapulpal placement of benzocaine gel (10-20%) followed by intrapulpal injection of local analgetic may be appropriate. Most of the analgesic effect is caused by pressure, so significant back pressure is necessary. Little analgesia is obtained by flooding the chamber.

Nitrous oxide (30-50% with oxygen) may be a significant aid to pain control. The patient must first be taught to breathe through the nose using a long, slow, deep paced cycle. Oral drugs, such as diazepam or barbiturates, are of little benefit here as their course is unpredictable. In the most difficult of management situations, intravenous medications should be considered. In this situation, diazepam or midazolam with or without methohexital, may be indicated.

Canals should be instrumented completely with care to avoid perforating the apex. If significant swelling is present and the tooth does not spontaneously drain, do an extracoronal incision and drainage. There is much debate about triphination of the apex, and the trend is to move away from this procedure as in many cases it further complicates the postoperative period.

Canals should be debrided using dilute sodium hypochloride and sterile saline or water. After drying, 0.1 ml dexamethasone (4 mg/ml) may be injected in the canal and pumped into place using a file. Steroids have been suggested to reduce postoperative pain. There is also some evidence for the use of calcium hydroxide powder mixed with saline or sterile water as a canal medicament.

The use of CMCP (camphor paramonochlorophenol), and formocresol is irritating to apical tissues and is not recommended.

Although there remains some debate on this issue, most experts recommend that teeth be sealed after treament. In the presence of swelling, the extracoronal incision and drainage should relieve any pressure. Leaving teeth open results in superinfection with oral microorganisms and contributes to a stormier postoperative course.

Analgesics and warm rinses should be continued in the postoperative period. The patient's condition should be reviewed in 24 hours. If necessary, reopen the tooth, irrigate, and reseal the access.

Periodontal diseases

Pain associated with the diagnosis and treatment of periodontal conditions appears to be one of the reasons only a minority of patients seek and follow through with care.

Examination

In patients with significant gingival inflammation and those with periodontitis, the gingival tissues often are quite sensitive to probing. While radiographs cannot replace probing, early and judicious use of both can minimize pain. This approach will produce the ultimate goal getting more patients to follow through with treatment. Often more extensive probings can be done using topical and injected local analgetics at the time of initial therapy.

Prophylaxis

Even in uncomplicated cases of gingivitis, scaling can be painful. Patients should be offered the use of topical analgesia and injected local analgesia even when the trauma of care seems minimal to the clinician. This approach is especially important when a dental auxilliary provides the care and the dentist may be unaware of the pain control problem. The dentist should discuss pain control with the patient at the initial consultation. Consideration also should be given to dividing treatment over two visits to reduce discomfort.

Soft tissue procedures

These procedures may include closed flap curettage and uncomplicated flap procedures. Even though these procedures are the least likely of the periodontal procedures to cause significant postoperative pain, 50% of patients do report pain. Careful consideration should be given to reducing inflammation and bacterial growth before surgical treatment. Strategies employing a one- to two-weeks course of tetracycline HCl (250 mg q.i.d.) or equivalent and twice daily rinses with chlorhexidine gluconate 0.12% or 0.2% may result in less overall trauma. A single dose of acetaminophen (1000 mg) or ibuprofen (400-600 mg) taken one hour before the procedure also may be helpful.

Osseous surgery and mucogingival procedures

These procedures are 3.5 to 6 times more likely to produce significant postoperative pain than are soft tissue procedures. Pain control should begin with a preoperative dose of ibuprofen (400-600 mg) taken 1 hour before surgery. If the patient cannot tolerate nonsteroidal drugs, acetaminophen can be substituted.

Local analgesia procedures should be performed carefully and slowly to reduce pain of injection. Some authors have suggested that long-acting local analgetics with vasoconstrictors may provide better analgesia to reduce postoperative pain problems in periodontal surgery: 0.5% bupivacaine with epinephrine 1:200,000 is suggested. However, surgery using this drug resulted in greater bleeding than in the comparison group using 2% lidocaine, 1:100,000 epinephrine. Others have proposed using intraseptal injections using a periodontal ligament syringe as an effective alternative to field blocks and supraperiosteal infiltrations. In this technique, single injections are made in the interdental papillae on the buccal and lingual 2 mm below the top of the papilla. The injection is 45 degrees to the long axis of the tooth. Lidocaine 2% with 1:50,000 epinephrine and a 27-gauge short needle is used. The main reason for considering this procedure as an alternative to conventional analgesia is the absence of the traditional lip or tongue numbness and similar side effects. Also less solution is needed, reducing potential toxicity. On the other hand, careful inspection of the data shows that 48% of patients reported pain on injection and 22% reported pain or discomfort during surgical procedures. There were no significant side effects reported.

Postoperative discomfort is significantly related to the duration of surgery. Therefore, it may be advantageous to limit the duration of the surgical procedure when possible, or divide the treatment in two more visits.

Patients who receive periodontal packs reportedly experience more discomfort. Alternatives may be to use antibiotics or chlorhexidine rinses following surgery.

Suprofen (200-400 mg), and ibuprofen (200-400 mg) are fairly effective in controlling pain and inflammation after periodontal surgery. Because peak plasma levels of these drugs occur one to two hours after administration, a preoperative dose is recommended. All of these drugs may have side effects and maximal doses should be carefully observed.

Treatment of periodontal abscesses

If at all possible, acute abscesses should initially be managed pharmacologically. That is, reduce symptoms with antibiotics, irrigate with chlorhexidine, and give analgesics before treating the local periodontal infection. This approach will increase the possibility that analgesia will be effective, and may reduce postoperative pain. When the problem is explored locally, complications such as endodontic involvement or fractured roots should be ruled out.

Dental hypersensitivity

Among the most common clinical problems faced by dentists caring for adult patients are complaints of pain in the cervical areas of the teeth. For many patients the reassurance that the problem is not caries or other infection is appropriate management. For others further steps are needed.

There are two major theories about the source of the pain. The first postulates that the pain is a result of the hydrodynamic forces expressed via exposed dentinal tubules. The second theory argues that pulpal sensory nerve activity results from pulpal inflammation.

Tooth brushing slowly removes the dentin smear layer in exposed areas of cementum. Extracted teeth that were sensitive before extraction show eight-fold increases in open tubules and larger tubule diameters. The most common sites for pain are on the buccal surfaces, especially in the upper jaw. The fluid in open tubules is postulated to serve as a transducer mechanism in the stimulation of nerve fibers in the pulp-dentin interface. Also, plaque may contain toxins that diffuse into the pulp and cause inflammation.

Most treatments proposed today follow the hydrodynamic theory and attempt to block or occlude the open tubules. The tooth has natural defenses and recovery occurs spontaneously in many cases, perhaps from reparative dentin or sclerotic dentin formation or mineralization of acquired pellicle. Recovery also may result from intratubule crystal formation, adsorption of plasma proteins to the inner surface of the tubules, or development of a smear layer. Consistent with the smear layer hypothesis, researchers have found that burnishing NaF/kaolin/glycerin paste into the root surface with an orangewood stick reduced dentin permeability but that the burnishing process was quite painful.

Treatments of root surfaces with oxalate salts produces crystal of calcium oxalate capable of occluding tubules and reducing sensitivity. The tooth surface is first dried and repeated applications are necessary with drying in between. Ordinary toothpaste containing fume silica as an abrasive also can deposit crystals to block tubules. The paste can be used as a topical agent, applied with a finger. Some data from research on cats suggest potassium-containing agents might be effective in reducing sensitivity.

Researchers recently have compared the effect of

0.42% sodium fluoride/ 3.96% strontium chloride (Lorric) with photocurring dentin bonding agent (Scotchbond). Although only a pilot study, the data suggest some promise for the bonding agent. Also 15-20% of teeth were not effectively desensitized with bonding. Little is known about any side effects regarding pulpal inflammation from the bonding treatment. Similarly a fluoride dentifrice (Protest-F) was ineffective in treating dentin sensitivity when used up to four months.

In a study comparing a dentifrice containing 10% strontium chloride (Sensodyne) with placebo 55% of test subjects reported total relief of subjective symptoms after 12 weeks versus only 14% of placebo subjects. Test subjects also reported some improvement in thermal sensitivity, but no change in tactile sensitivity.

Recommendations regarding changes in diet and the importance of oral cleanliness also may be helpful in reducing dentinal pain.

Concerns related to restorative dentistry

Another tooth-sensitivity problem is related to dental cements. Previous work suggested that zinc phosphate cements could cause a transient pulpal inflammation and pain. Recently concerns have been raised about carboxylate and glass ionomer cements. Both use polyacrylic acid as a bonding medium. Apparently the polycarboxylate agents generate little pulpal response because they incorporate zinc powder.

There is considerable potential advantage to using the glass ionomer cements in restorative dentistry because of their bonding to metal and tooth and their release of fluoride from the silicate component. One preliminary clinical study examined the postcementation responses to glass ionomer cement with crowns in place for six months. It suggests relatively few problems occurred; the results were little different than with zinc phosphate. However, such studies are preliminary, not well controlled, and do not entirely eliminate concern.

At least two approaches are being tried to reduce potential problems. Some authors have suggested that resin-compatible cavity varnishes reduce dentin permeability *in vitro*. Any of the popular products (e.g., nitrocellulose based or polyamide) are acceptable. The second approach advocates the use of potassium oxalate to close dentin tubules to the insult of polyacrylic acid from the filling material. This approach did not lower bond strengths of zinc phosphate or polycarboxylate cements, but increased the bond strength of glass ionomer cement.

Selected problems with oral soft tissues

Denture sore mouth and candidiasis

Bacterial and fungal infections have been suggested as the cause of these painful problems. Cleaning and disinfecting the denture with dilute sodium hypochloride, or chlorhexidine is helpful; the patient should remove the denture overnight. Some of these problems, such as burning mouth, may have natural periods of spontaneous remission. Over-the-counter rinses such as Listerine or denture soaks such as Efferdent may help. Treatment with antifungal agents, such as nystatin or clotrimazole, also may be needed in some cases.

Oral mucositis

Patients undergoing chemotherapy, especially for leukemia, experience very painful and prolonged mucositis. Two approaches have been advocated: diphenhydramine rinses and chlorhexidine gluconate 0,12% rinses. Both approaches seem to reduce the duration and severity of the pain.

Herpetic lesions

As yet there are no agents that eliminate the virus, so treatment is limited to symptomatic relief. The basic strategy is lubrication, ice chips, bland diet, viscous lidocaine or benzocaine in orabase for discrete lesions, and systemic analgesics. In particularly uncomfortable cases a linguet of methyl testostone may be recommended. Similarly, a rinse of elexir of diphenhydramine and milk of magnesia is useful.

Oral lichen planus

These lesions do not require treatment if asymptomatic. If painful, try injecting corticosteroids directly into the lesion or using a corticosteroid cream with/or without a celluloid base preparation.

Alveolitis sicca dolorosa

This condition (ASD) usually is termed a "dry socket", as the blood clot normally produced in an extraction socket disappears. The process is thought to be caused by fibrinolysis of the coagulum, probably induced by an infection of the clot and the alveolar socket with anerobic microorganisms, hence the foul taste and smell. Also, other factors, such as traumatic surgery are believed to play a role.

ASD can be avoided by administering an antibiotic before surgery. Investigations have shown that both penicillin and metronidazole are effective in preventing ASD. Normally, 0.5 g of metronidazole a half-hour before surgery is recommended in all cases of lower third molar removal. A one-time dosage protects the clot for several days postoperatively. It is of little or no use to prescribe antibiotics postoperatively, as the clot has no blood supply until granulation tissue develops after 2-3 days. It is, therefore, important to administer the antibiotic before surgery.

Acute pericoronitis predisposes to ASD. When a tooth is extracted in an acute stage of infection, the patient should be given 4 mill units (or 3 g) of penicillin V before surgery. If the patient is allergic to penicillin, 1 g of metronidazole is recommended. If the patient's immune apparatus is compromised e.g., treatment with systemic glucocorticosteroids or cytotoxic drugs, leukemia, or bone marrow depression, but not diabetes mellitus), it is advisable to continue the antibiotic coverage for 3-4 days postoperatively.

Preoperative rinsing of the oral cavity with 0.2% chlorhexidine, followed by postoperative rinsing twice daily with a 0.1% solution of chlorhexidine is very effective in reducing the risk of ASD. Postoperative rinse with the 0.1% solution reduces the incidence of chlorhexidine side effects such as metallic taste, discoloration of teeth and mucous membrane, and epithelial desquamation.

A patient with ASD typically experiences a foul or rotten taste in the mouth, and increasingly strong pain with irradiation to the ear. Fibrinolysis and the infection in the socket trigger the local production of bradykinin, an algogenic or pain-producing peptide. Clinically, the socket is empty, and detritus can be removed easily by irrigation.

Treatment of ASD

The socket is carefully irrigated with one of the following solutions:

- physiologic saline
- 0.2% chlorhexidine
- 1.5% hydrogen peroxide.

Then the socket is packed loosely with a small gauze strip moistened with eugenol or tincture of benzoin to give immediate pain relief. The pack should be removed after 24 hours, and the socket thoroughly irrigated with one of the above-mentioned solutions. The socket should not be packed again, as the pack will inhibit the normal healing processes, and thus prolong the condition. To remain pain free, the patient should irrigate the socket whenever pain occurs. Give the patient instructions on how to use a 10 ml syringe and an irrigation needle. This method relieves the pain as irrigation removes the precursors of bradykinin and prostaglandins. Pain persisting after one week should raise a suspicion of necrosis and sequestrum formation; surgical exploration of the area is indicated.

Ostitis sicca
(pain following root-canal therapy)

This very painful condition arises in the apical area during or after a root canal treatment. It is thought to be caused by either a mechanical stimulation of the area as the root canal reamer is pressed out of the apical foramen, or by a chemical irritation if the disinfecting solution used to cleanse the canal is forced out into the same region. Sometimes the facial bone plate is very thin or even missing, so the very sensitive periosteum is directly stimulated. The patient usually experiences a rather sharp, well-localized pain in the periapical region. This condition is most often incorrectly diagnosed as an infection, and then unsuccessfully attempted being treated with antibiotics.

Treatment of ostitis sicca

The best way to treat this condition is to remove any medicament in the root canal, and then carefully administer soluble dexamethasone on a paper point. The same drug can be injected in the soft tissues opposite the painful tooth after local analgesia has been obtained. Dexamethasone is available in many parts of the world premixed with lidocaine. Some experts recommend administering 4 mg dexamethasone IM followed by daily oral doses. An analgesic also should be prescribed, but antibiotics are given only in the case of obvious signs of infection.

Periostitis

As the name suggests, this condition is an inflammation of the periosteum, usually very painful due to the high content of pain nociceptors in this layer. It is caused most often by a traumatic condition, as suggested above, or bad surgery that unduly traumatizes the periosteum. Another cause of periostitis can be bone or tooth particles left after surgical intervention, especially following removal of impacted third molars. Before the periosteal flap is sutured, it is very important to irrigate the socket and beneath the flap with physiologic saline.

Treatment of periostitis

Antibiotics usually are the treatment of choice, combined with local wound care and irrigation with 1.5% hydrogen peroxide. If an abscess has formed under the periosteum (bone-hard, very tender swelling), it should be drained by incision or by opening the suture line.

Sinusitis

Infection of the maxillary sinus often will result in pain or ache in the posterior teeth on the same side. Acute sinusitis is characterized by severe throbbing pain, swelling, toothache, and unilateral drainage from the nostril on the affected side. About 40% of all infections in the maxillary sinus are odontogenic in origin, apical periodontitis, and deep marginal involvement, and they usually are caused by anerobic microorganisms. Other reasons for sinusitis include infection from the nose through the ostium, or allergic reactions in the mucous membrane of the sinus. Viruses certainly play a role. Dry air also can worsen the condition as the cilia function in the sinus is impaired with ensuing stasis of mucus.

Treatment of sinusitis

Acute sinusitis requires antibiotic treatment. Penicillin V is the drug of choice, as 2 mill units (1.5 g) b.i.d. for 3-4 days. When the infection is odontogenic, metronidazole is very effective, administered as 0.5 g t.i.d. for 3-4 days. Decongesting nasal drops are advocated, e.g., ephedrine 1% 3-4 times daily. The patient should not use the drops for longer than a week, or a secondary rebound hyperemia might develop.

In case of chronic sinusitis with postnasal drip, inhalation of a mist of lukewarm saline is recommended together with a decongestant. Antibiotics are rarely indicated for chronic sinusitis. The causative factor should be traced and removed if possible.

Dysesthesia of the inferior alveolar and lingual nerves

Any damage to a nerve can result in decreased function and nerve pain (i.e., neuralgia). If the damage causes inflammation or infection in the nerve, the condition is called a *neuritis*.

Three terms require definition:

1. *Anesthesia* means "without feeling at all", and follows a direct severing of the nerve, be it chemical, surgical, or traumatic. The patient will have no feeling in the affected area.
2. *Paresthesia* means a feeling of numbness and tingling in the area. It is not completely dead, and occasionally the patient has a sense of feeling in the affected area, much like the sensation that returns following a local analgesia.
3. *Dysesthesia* means that the "feeling is wrong". Patients usually will complain of a paresthetic feeling with increased hypersensibility to touch or function. An elec-

tric shock sensation might occur. Dysesthesia usually is the worst of these three conditions, which are all signs of nerve damage. In most cases the nerve will regenerate, that is the proximal stump will sprout and follow the perineurium (the Schwann's sheath) of the distal stump. The regeneration normally will begin after one month, during which a degeneration takes place (the Wallerian degeneration). If the sprouting process succeeds, the regenerating nerve will grow 1 mm per day until it reaches its terminal branches. A beginning sensation of "life" is called Tinel's sign.

Damage to the *inferior alveolar nerve*, which most frequently happens after surgical removal of the lower third molar, will disturb sensation in the lower lip. This problem also can occur after surgery in the mental foramen region. This sensation bothers patients who often feel that saliva or fluid, when they drink, will leak out the corner of the mouth and down on the lip and the chin. They may constantly wipe off the lip with a handkerchief or napkin. In most cases the patient can be comforted and told that there is a 95% chance that normal sensation will return in one year. Little can be done to improve the situation. When an amputation neuroma is suspected, the bone canal can be opened by a sagittal split osteotomy, and the damaged nerve repaired with a sural nerve transplantation under microscope.

If damage to the inferior alveolar nerve is suspected before surgery to occur due to an anatomic close relation between the mandibular canal and the root tip, *it is very important to inform the patient about the risk of sensational disturbances*. This information also should be noted in the patient's record. If the patient does not want the surgery, then don't do it. Many legal cases have resulted from poor information and bad recording in the charts.

Damage to the *lingual nerve* unfortunately is more permanent than to the inferior alveolar nerve, the difference probably being that the lingual nerve lies in the soft tissues, while the inferior alveolar nerve lies in a bony canal to facilitate regenerative growth. Lingual nerve dysfunction includes a loss of taste on the ipsilateral side of the tongue.

In some cases of lingual nerve damage persisting for more than six months, it is advisable to do an exploratory operation lingual to the third molar region, where the original damage most likely was inflicted. In some cases, a band of tight scar tissue binds the nerve down to the sharp mylohyoid line. Loosening of this band sometimes will allow return of normal sensation. If the nerve is severed during an operation and this is discovered immediately, the two nerve ends should be sutured at once. In any case, nerve damage with following sensational dysfunction is always an unhappy situation for both the patient and the dentist.

Trigeminal nerve neuralgia

Neuralgia means a throbbing, sharp pain, often occurring in attacks along a nerve. *Typical* trigeminal neuralgia (tic douloureux) is characterized by very intense, burning stabbing pain attacks in one, two, or even all three trigeminal branches. The attacks usually are elicited by stimulating a certain trigger zone by touch, eating, shaving, and so forth. The attacks last for a few minutes, followed by pain-free intervals.

Atypical trigeminal neuralgia is characterized by the same type of pain, although not of the same intensity, and the attacks normally will last for half an hour or longer. Some researchers believe that this type of pain is caused by dysfunction in the muscles of mastication. A pain or suffering that is constant although variable in character is never a genuine trigeminal neuralgia.

Many theories have been put forward to explain trigeminal neuralgia. Two of the more realistic ones point to:

1. *The short-circuit theory.* It is thought that the myelin

sheath surrounding all larger nerve fibers can degenerate and disappear, especially in the semilunar ganglion. This condition creates an area of increased risk for shortcircuiting the impulses, thus spreading from a few nerves to many nerves. The reason for this myelin degeneration is not known, but it is speculated that virus might be responsible.

2. *The vascular compression theory.* Many blood vessels are passing the semilunar ganglion area, close to the internal carotid and the sinus cavernosus. Vascular dysfunction is thought to compress the ganglion and cause the pain attacks.

Treatment of trigeminal neuralgia

The most accepted treatment of typical trigeminal neuralgia is to administer carbamazepine. This drug originally was developed as an antiepileptic and is still used as such. It is believed to stabilize the surface membrane of hyperexcitable nerve tissue. Carbamazepine will relieve typical trigeminal neuralgia in 80-90% of cases. If the effect is less than desirable, it can be combined with, or substituted by phenytoin and diazepam. If medical treatment is insufficient, injection of glycerol into the cisterne surrounding the trigeminal ganglion can be attempted. Another possibility is electrocoagulation of sensible areas of the ganglion, using stereoscopic X ray to guide the needle. Some success has been claimed with cryosurgery of the infraorbital or mental nerves.

Cutting the nerves (exhairesis) or alcohol or phenol injections are not recommended today. Destroying nerve tissue can lead to the uncomfortable situation of anesthesia dolorosa, i.e., pain in an anesthestic area. Even though the afferent nerve has been cut, the pain feeling can return; other nerve tracts able to conduct pain seem to be activated.

Post-herpetic neuralgia

Following a herpetic infection, some patients develop a dreadful condition called herpes zoster which features very intense burning pain on one side of the body. This condition is very difficult to treat, and many cases do not respond. In the early stages, sympathetic blocks can be attempted. Later on in the course, TENS or acupuncture have sometimes proven helpful. In severe cases, alpha-adrenergic blocking agents such as phentolamine can be tried.

Cluster headache

Other terms for cluster headache are migrainous headache or periodic migrainoid neuralgia. It most often affects active males 40-60 years old. Typically, symptoms are severe burning, throbbing or toothache-like, unilateral pain, occurring in several attacks at nighttime. The patients will wake up because of the pain, and find the nose blocked and the eye injected on the ipsilateral side. Histamine release may be responsible for at least some of the symptoms, and therefore, the condition also is known as a histamine headache.

Treatment is the same as for classic migraine, i.e., ergotamines. Antihistamines and antiserotonines also can be tried.

Classic migraine

Classic migraine differs from common migraine as the former condition begins with a prodromal phase (aura) characterized by dizziness, scotoma (light flashes), weakness, nausea, and vomiting. Then follows a very severe unilateral throbbing headache, caused by a vasodilation of cerebral vessels. Common migraine has the same type of pain, but no prodromal phase or aura. Many researchers believe that the common migraine is the same condition as acute myofascial pain syndrome involving the temporalis muscle.

Treatment of migraine

The acute attack is most frequently treated with ergotamine (a vasoconstrictor). Another current symptomatic treatment is the combination of 1 g of acetylsalicylic acid plus 10 mg of diazepam and 10 mg of metoclopramide; all three can be administered rectally. The patient is then allowed to sleep for 12-24 hours.

In some cases migraine can be prevented by drugs such as methysergide, clonidine, cyproheptadine, pizotiphen, and beta-blocking agents.

References

1. Addy M. Aetiology, oral distribution and management of dentine hypersensitivity. IADR Abstract No 549, March 1987.

2. Balaban FS, Skidmore AE, Griffin JA. Acute exacerbations following initial treatment of necrotic pulps. J Endod Feb 1984; 10(2): 78-81.

3. Bell WE. Orofacial pains: Classification, diagnosis, and management. 3rd ed. Chicago: Year Book Medical Publishers, Inc., 1985.

4. Birn H. Etiology and pathogenesis of fibrinolytic alveolitis. Int J Oral Surg 1973; 2: 211-63.

5. Curtis JW, McLain JB, Hutcheson RA. The incidence and severity of complications and pain following periodontal surgery. J Periodontol Oct. 1985; 56(10): 597-660.

6. Genet JM, Wesselink PR, Thoden Van Velzen SK. The incidence of preoperative and postoperative pain in endodontic therapy. In Endod J 1986; 19: 22-229.

7. Johnson WT, Leary JM. Vertical root fractures: diagnosis and treatment. General Dentistry Sept-Oct 1984; pp 425-29.

8. Krasner P, Jackson E. Management of post-treatment endodontic pain with oral dexamethasone: a double blind study. Oral Surg 1986; 62(2): 187-190.

9. MacGregor AF, Addy A. Value of penicillin in the prevention of pain, swelling and trismus following the removal of ectopic mandibular third molars. Int J Oral Surg 1980; 9: 166-72.

10. Moore PA. Bupivacaine: a long-lasting local anesthetic for dentistry. Oral Surg 1984; 58(4): 369-73.

11. Pashley DH. Treatment of dentin sensitivity through tubule occlusion. IADR Abstract No 546, March 1987.

12. Petersen JK. Diflunisal, a new analgesic in the treatment of postoperative pain following removal of impacted mandibular third molars. Int J Oral Surg 1979; 8: 102-13.

13. Rodgers RS III (ed.) Disorders of mucous membranes. Dermatologic clinica vol 5(4), Oct. 87.

14. Rood, JP, Murgatroyd J. Metronidazole in the prevention of dry socket. Br J Oral Surg 1979; 17: 62-70.

15. Rud J. Third molar surgery. Relationship of root to mandibular canal and injuries to inferior dental nerve. Tandlægebladet 1983; 87: 619-31.

16. Rud J. Third molar surgery. Perforation of the inferior dental nerve through the root. Tandlægebladet 1983; 87: 659-67.

17. Seymour RA, Walton JG. Pain control after third molar surgery. Int J Oral Surg 1984; 13: 457-85.

18. Vogel RI, Grop JI. The effects of nonsteroidal antiinflammatory analgesics on pain after periodontal surgery. JADA 1984; 109: 731-34.

19. Wessberg GA, Wolford LM, Epker B. Simultaneous inferior alveolar nerve graft and osseous reconstruction of the mandible. J Oral Maxillofac Surg 1982; 40: 384-90.

CHAPTER 12

Pain control in children

Pain control for children generally follows the same principles as for adults. This chapter highlights major areas of importance. Several conceptual issues first need clarification. One, pain generally is underrecognized and often not treated in children, especially in very young ones. Recent research has suggested the need to be more sensitive to pain in children.

Second, pain is a key factor in the development of fear. Our recent research finds that over 200 persons per thousand express high dental fear. Injections rank high on the lists of feared stimuli, and most high-fear persons report their fear developed in childhood. Most of this fear resulted from early restorative dentistry experiences, which makes prevention of caries disease most important.

Finally the concept of control is essential to avoid traumatizing children. Control is instilled using behavioral strategies ranging from tell-show-do to signalling and behavioral rehearsals. These approaches are part of a model of directed guidance of child behavior demonstrated to be most successful in clinic research and practice. This same research ample shows the negative consequences and ineffectiveness of aversive child management techniques such as the hand-over-mouth strategy. Such abusive approaches, although taught for many years, are inappropriate and should not be used. For a review of appropriate strategies see *Treating Dental Patients: A Patient Management Handbook*.

Behavioral techniques

Powerful behavioral strategies such as distraction (discussed in Chapter 4) are equally effective in school-age

97

children. Distraction is most efficacious when pain is of short duration and intensity. Asking the child to watch a favorite TV program in his or her mind or to imagine a favorite activity works well.

Other strategies include having the child listen to a favorite audio tape or even telling the child a story. The more captivating distractor will work the best.

Nitrous oxide at levels of approximately 30% with oxygen is analgesic with children. Research suggests nitrous oxide is most effective when it is combined with sound behavioral strategies. A clinician skilled in using behavioral techniques is better than a poor one using nitrous oxide alone. Introduce the child to the use of nitrous oxide at an early appointment prior to sessions for restorative work, so the child can briefly practice the required behaviors of slow paced breathing, relaxation, and distraction. Never use nitrous oxide when local analgesia already has been given and proved ineffectual or when a child is out of control or hysterical.

Injections

Good technique is essential for painless and effective analgesia with children. Topical analgesia should always be employed. Ethylaminobenzoate (benzocaine) or similar drugs, usually in the ointment form, are effective. They have rapid onset (1-2 minutes) and fairly long duration. They also have very limited toxicity or allergy potential. These viscous materials can be applied on a cotton roll left in a place or on a cotton swab. Use caution to avoid the topical getting everywhere and alarming the child. Similarly, liquids and sprays are difficult to control. Also, taste the preparation yourself to avoid unpleasant materials.

There is much clinical lore about painless injections. The key factors appear to be topical analgesia, blanching pressure on the tissue and slow, where possible, careful injection. A rate of 1 ml per minute is appropriate. Most

Table 4
Maximum recommended drug dosages

Drug	w/o vasoconstrictor mg/kg	w/ vasoconstrictor mg/kg
Lidocaine	4.4	7.0
Mepivacaine	6.6	6.6
Prilocaine	7.9	7.9

dentists need to time themselves to learn to proceed that slowly.

Most analgesia in the primary dentition can be accomplished using infiltration/or supraperiosteal technique. Only extensive restorative or endodontic procedures require more extensive block injections. On the other hand, by the time a child reaches adolescence, cortical bone has become so dense that an approach appropriate for an adult is needed.

There is little difference in approaching children and adults. A key exception is for the inferior alveolar block (mandibular block). Anatomical studies find the child's mandibular foramen to be slightly below the occlusal plane.

For children weighing over about 100 pounds (45 kg), dosages of local analgetics are essentially the same as for adults. Maximum recommended dosages are given in Table 4.

It is essential to aspirate before injecting in the oral cavity - 25 to 27 gauge needles and intraligamentary injections can be used in children as a substitute or adjunct to conventional technique. Use 2% lidocaine with 1: 50,000 epinephrine. This approach is especially useful as an adjunct with endodontic procedures. Intraligamentary injections also avoid the discomfort of soft tissue anesthesia and prevent inadvertent cheek chewing or lip biting in small children. There also is some evidence that placing benzocaine ointment on an exposed pulp may

99

Table 5	
Acetaminophen doses for children	
Age/years	Dose/mg
under 1	60
1-6	60-120
6-12	150-300

produce temporary analgesia and perhaps allow access for intrapulpal injection.

Postoperative pain management with children

In children, 90% of pain episodes can be managed with acetaminophen or aspirin. Generally, acetaminophen is recommended because of its lower toxicity. Table 5 gives dosing guidelines for acetaminophen.

Single dose every 4-6 hours not exceed 1.2 g/day.

Aspirin divided over 4-5 doses can be given at 65 mg/kg. Aspirin should not be given to children with flu-like symptoms because of concerns over Reyes Syndrome, or to children below the age of 2 years.

Other pain problems with children

Teething

About 60% of children who are teething will exhibit irritability, restlessness, drooling, disturbed sleep, rash, fever, or diarrhea. In most cases, pain medication is not appropriate. Rather, a chewable object and a lubricant for the chapped skin is best. If pain and fever are a problem, acetaminophen and judicious use of topical analgesia may be considered; rule out infection.

Pain of herpetic or similar lesions

Management of these self-limiting conditions should include bland diets and acetaminophen as needed. Surface protectants may have limited utility. A local analgesic rinse of viscous lidocaine, Kaopectate 50% - Benylin 50% also may be used. If pain persists and the patient exhibits malaise, consider systemic injection and promptly refer the child to a pediatrician.

Bruxism-TMJ-Headache in children

There is considerable evidence that children experience muscle tenderness and soreness of teeth on biting because of bruxism. In one study 33% of school-age children reported pain. One researcher reports that 15-23% of a sample of adolescents in the US have recurrent headache. Another researcher reported TMJ pain in 0.7-2.0% of a sample of over 2000 Japanese school children. Neither of these samples is completely representative and little data exist to allow generalization. Nonetheless, there is some basis for saying that such pain is experienced by some children

Recommended treatment is symptomatic, employing behavioral techniques such as relaxation, biofeedback, and reassurance. Vapocoolants such as ethyl chloride or a soft splint may be helpful.

References

1. Bennett CR. Local anesthetic considerations in pediatric dental patients, Chapter 19 in Braham R, Morris M. (eds.) Textbook of Pediatric Dentistry, 2nd ed. Baltimore: Williams & Wilkins, 1985.
2. Peterson RG. Antipyretics and analgesics in children. Der Pharmacol Ther 1985; 8: 68-84.

CHAPTER 13

Pain control in the elderly patient

The pain control problems in the elderly focus on general and prosthetic dentistry, oral medicine, and oral surgery.

General dentistry

Pulp size, dentin deposits, and vascularity of teeth change with normal aging. Dentin continues to be deposited throughout life while the amount of pulp tissue decreases. Vascularity decreases markedly and evidence suggests that the aging pulp has less ability to respond to noxious stimuli especially agents permeating through the dentin. This change may presage increased endodontic and periodontic lesions in the elderly, who now retain a larger proportion of their teeth.

There has been much scientific debate about pain threshold and pain tolerance in the elderly. Results of direct investigations of pain threshold suggest no difference in younger and older patients. That is, elderly patients feel pain from a pulp tester in their teeth the same as do younger individuals. Thus, the automatic assumption that older patients do not need local analgesia may be incorrect. Such beliefs about the pain perception of the elderly stemmed from extrapolating from the findings of skin burn tests that have little relevance to the teeth.

There is evidence, on the other hand, that the ability to discriminate between levels of suprathreshold pain changes. Elderly persons may report low-grade pain as more painful than that reported by younger individuals. Pain tolerance (e.g., the level at which pain becomes too great for drilling) is related to cultural factors and experience rather than clear physiological sensory differences. Complaints of pain also may relate to depression and other psychosomatic problems. Nonetheless, each patient should be evaluated individually.

Local analgesia is preferred for operative pain control. Any amide agent may be used; all will be equally effective in most situations. The use of ester type drugs should be evaluated carefully in view of possible drug interactions/ and decreased pseudocholinesterases. The dose of local analgetics should not exceed 9 ml of 2% lidocaine or similar drugs. Similarly the amount of epinephrine used as a vasoconstrictor should be limited to 0.04 mg in patients with organic heart disease, and avoided entirely in patients with hyperthyroidism, those taking monoamine oxidase inhibitors, adrenergic blockers, or tricyclic antidepressants. Instead use 3% mepivacaine or prilocaine.

Careful anesthetic technique is required for all patients, but especially in the elderly. The amide linkage is metabolized primarily by liver microsomal enzymes, which may not function as well in the elderly as in younger persons. Thus, toxic overdose through vascular injection (with failure to aspirate during injection) is a risk.

Prosthetic dentistry and oral medicine

Several potentially painful conditions are associated with dentures. Among the most common are angular cheilosis, epulis fissuratum, and denture stomatitis. Surveys show that over 60% of the elderly will be taking one or more over-the-counter agents so a careful history is necessary. Treatment of these conditions involves identifying the cause, such as an overclosed vertical dimension or candida infection, and treating it appropriately.

Recently, some researchers reported that several over-the-counter products were effective in reducing plaque levels associated with denture stomatitis, even in the absence of mechanical denture hygiene. Groups rinsed daily three times and used overnight soaks. A combination of Listerine rinses and soaks with Efferdent proved effective clinically. Listerine also was effective with overnight soaks of sterile water.

Oral surgery

Often recovery in the elderly is prolonged over that in younger individuals. Use smaller, more frequent dosings of analgesics for the postoperative pain associated with endodontics and periodontics as well as for extractions or preprosthetic surgery. Just as in oral surgery with younger individuals, a presurgery loading dose is appropriate.

In the United States, 40% of the elderly take one or more analgesic preparations each day. Therefore, the clinician needs to be sensitive to potential overdose toxicity and drug interactions. Experts point out that aspirin and acetaminophen (paracetamol) with or without codeine are prescribed most often for dental pain. They suggest acetaminophen (500-600 mg) is effective and avoids the complications involved in aspirin use by the elderly.

Combining acetaminophen with codeine is only slightly more efficacious, and for many individuals adds significant side effects from its CNS activity. Ibuprofen (200-400 mg) is efficacious but can produce drowsiness, dizziness, stomatitis, and vertigo in some individuals. Effectiveness plateau is at 200-400 mg in the elderly, higher doses are not more effective.

Other narcotics analgesics generally are contraindicated for dental pain in elderly patients. Such drugs depress respiration and circulation.

In prescribing pain control drug for the elderly patients, give written directions. All patients should be urged to rest after dental procedures: sedative agents also may be appropriate at one-half the dose used in younger patients.

Reference

1. Tryon AF, (ed.) Oral health and aging. Littleton, MA: PSG Publishing Co. Inc., 1986.

CHAPTER 14

Information for patients

Patients generally perceive that dentists are insensitive to the pain they feel. With such patients it is often helpful for the dentist to discuss pain and pain control. Begin by asking about previous dental visits. Was pain control adequate? Is there anything special you want me to do? These questions will yield valuable information.

Pain is a personal, subjective experience that may or may not involve obvious tissue damage. The dentist's first responsibility is to be empathic. Never deny a patient's view of previous experiences. Rather, accept these views and plan your approach accordingly. If pain control is inadequate, it is the fault of the dentist not the patient.

Pain control should be explained as a joint responsibility of the patient and dentist. The patient should try to relax and breathe calmly to reduce the muscle tension that is the source of much pain. The patient also can use self-distraction or another strategy. The dentist must be effective and thorough in using local analgesics.

Patient concerns about local analgesia

Explain to the patient the steps being taken to make injections comfortable. A demonstration of the effectiveness of topical analgesia may help. Some patients need reassurance that the entire length of the needle won't be used. For those who fear the injection itself, desensitization, described in Chapter 4, is helpful.

Some patients may be concerned about reactions to local analgetics. Never deny or make light of these fears. Rather, attempt to understand them. Take a two-step approach to these concerns. First, rule out allergy and toxicity. Patients may be skin tested, and careful history taking is invaluable. Toxicity reactions are rare. Second, rule out fear. Most often, psychophysiological reactions are the cause of problems. Patients often need careful explanations to grasp that the vasoconstrictors in local analgesics mimic natural drugs produced by the body. Other patients should be told about the numbness and loss of control associated with the analgesic.

Postoperative medications

Compliance is a major problem in controlling postoperative pain. Studies show only one-half of patients will actually purchase the drug and one-third will not take the drug according to directions. Your goal should be to reduce barriers to correct use of pain medications. Consider dispensing small quantities of drug rather than writing prescriptions. Have patients take initial doses at the office. A prescription can be provided for drugs needed beyond one day. However, the majority of patients will have little pain beyond one day.

Prescribe small doses of drugs at short intervals rather than longer ones. Use this strategy to keep a patient out of pain rather than instructing them to use a drug when pain occurs. The goal is to prevent pain. Use the drug least likely to cause side effects. Consider the nonsteroidal drugs before drugs containing codeine or other narcotics. Nausea, a common side effect of the narcotics, prompts patients to discontinue the pain control drug.

Use written instructions. Do not simply rely on the pharmacist to give instructions. A clear, simple set of instructions can be made up in advance and given to the patient. Discuss with the patient the need to call you if medications are inadequate to control pain. Be aware that many patients will self-medicate with over-the-counter of prescription drugs used for other medical problems or obtained from relatives.

Debriefing

Immediately after an operative procedure it's helpful to debrief the patient. Was pain control adequate? If it was not, you can reassure the patient that steps will be taken at the next appointment to control pain better. This simple step will greatly reduce appointments missed due to pain. Later in the day or evening after an appointment, a brief phone call from a staff member will be useful to ascertain that the patient is taking the medications as requested and is not experiencing any major problem.

CHAPTER 15

Temporomandibular disorders

Temporomandibular disorders (TMD) are a set of clinical problems involving pain in front of the ear and in related facial muscles, and limitations and deviations in jaw opening. This constellation of symptoms often is accompanied by audible joint sounds such as popping, clicking, or crepitus. This syndrome can be accompanied by other problems such as headache. Cognitive, affective, and psychosocial characteristics are potent predictors of TMD symptoms.

TMD is a major health problem and has been termed the most common and expanding disorder treated by dentists. Subjective pain is reported in 5-7% of the general population in many parts of the world; however it is very difficult to interpret and generalize from the many existing epidemiologic studies.

What causes TMD?

There are three major theories regarding the cause of this clinical problem: (1) bone and soft tissue pathology in the joint itself; (2) abnormal occlusion; and (3) muscle spasm, clenching, and bruxing. It has been argued that the disorder stems from psychological problems, stress, or secondary pain and illness behavior.

Some researchers suggest that personality factors and stress lead to muscle hyperactivity that eventually results in pain and limitations in mandibular movement. Others cite bruxism as the source of a muscular inflammatory response resulting in TMD. It seems likely, however, that TMD is determined by multiple interactive causes that involve neurological, psychosocial, and dental factors.

109

Data from the University of Washington clinics suggest the ratio for female to male clients with TM disorders is 5:2. It is not known whether this represents illness-seeking behavior or the actual underlying rate of disease. TMD patients generally are well educated. Seventeen percent of patients have had pain over 5 years, while 75 percent had developed pain in the last 12-24 months.

Treatment of TMD

It has been suggested that the pathologic cycle of this syndrome can be broken by directing therapy at three possible areas: occlusion, facial and masticatory muscles, or stress and tension. Most of the generally accepted therapies to the problem embody one of these approaches.

According to unpublished data the average patient received 5-6 different treatments over 5 months. Seventy percent received bite appliances. Other treatments commonly provided were: muscle or physical therapy (56%); analgesics or antiinflammatory agents, muscle relaxants, or psychoactive drugs (30%); or referral for counseling or stress reduction (28%). Surgery and/or occlusal adjustment was provided for only 2-4% patients. Pain was reduced in 67%, remained the same for 30%, and increased for 3%. These data are similar to much of the published treatment literature. They point to how little is known about the problem, and particularly to absence of data on the natural history of the untreated or underlying condition.

This area of clinical practice is plagued by uncontrolled, relatively asystematic reports of success from each clinic's approach. The various techniques employed are listed in Table 6.

It is generally agreed today that multiple conservative approaches using physiotherapy, muscle relaxants and analgesics, splints, and counseling form the bases of symptomatic therapy. Surgical approaches, whether joint surgery or dental reconstruction, are treatments used

	Table 6
	Treatments used in TM-disorders
Surgery	joint surgery
	muscle scarification
Pharmacological	muscle relaxants
	topical analgesics
	regional analgesics
	corticosteroids
	tranquilizers
Physiotherapy	heat
	exercise
	splints
Occlusal	spot grinding
	occlusal equilibration
	restorative dentistry
	prostheses
Psychological	psychotherapy
	counseling
	progressive relaxation

only after considerable efforts at conservative approaches have failed.

References

1. American Dental Association. Report of the President's Conference on the examination, diagnosis, and management of temporomandibular disorders. JADA 1983; 66: 75-77.
2. Dubner R, Sessle BJ, Storey AJ. The neural basis or oral and facial function. New York: Plenum Press, 1978.

3. Dworkin SF. A state of the sciences review: Major oro-facial pain syndromes. Paper prepared for NIDR, NIH, June 1982.

4. Rugh JD, Jacobs DT, et al. Psychophysiological changes and oral conditions, Chapter 1, in Cohen LK, Bryant PS (eds.) Social sciences and dentistry: A critical bibliography V.II. London: Federation Dentaire Internationale, 1984.

Glossary of terms

Allodynia

Pain due to a stimulus that normally does not provoke pain.

Analgesia

Absence of pain in response to stimulation that normally would be painful.

Analgesia, General

A condition, where pain sensation is more or less reduced, but consciousness and protective reflexes remain intact.

Analgesia, Local

A condition with temporarily suspended normal nerve transmission in a localized area of the body.

Analgesic

Pain relieving drug of either central or peripheral action.

Anesthesia

A condition where all sensations are suspended.

Anesthesia, General

A condition where all sensations, including consciousness, are temporarily suspended.

Anesthesia Dolorosa

Pain in area or region which is anesthetic.

Causalgia

A syndrome of sustained burning pain, allodynia, or hyperpathia after a traumatic nerve lesion, often combined with vasomotor and sudomotor dysfunction and later trophic changes.

Dysesthesia

An unpleasant abnormal sensation, whether spontaneous or evoked.

113

Endorphins	Endogenous produced morphine-like peptides that can reduce pain by inhibiting the release of substance P.
Gate Control	Pain reducing mechanism at the entrance of the posterior horn of the trigeminal tract nucleus or in the spinal medulla, involving the release of local endorphins.
Hyperesthesia	Increased sensitivity to stimulation, excluding the special senses.
Hyperalgesia	An increased response to a stimulus that normally is painful.
Hyperpathia	A painful syndrome, characterized by increased reaction to a stimulus, especially a repetitive stimulus as well as an increased threshold.
Hypoesthesia	Decreased sensitivity to stimulation, excluding the special senses.
Hypoalgesia	Diminished pain in response to a normally painful stimulus.
Neuralgia	Pain in the distribution of a nerve or nerves.
Neuritis	Inflammation of a nerve or nerves.
Neuropathy	A disturbance of function or pathological change in a nerve.
Nociceptor	A receptor preferentially sensitive to a noxious stimulus or to a stimulus that would be noxious if prolonged.
Pain	An unpleasant sensory and emotional experience associated with actual or potential tissue damage or described in terms of such damage.

Pain, Projected	A pain sensation that originates along a nerve fiber due to nerve fiber damage and results in pain in the normal distribution of that nerve.
Pain, Referred	A pain sensation that originates in one place but is felt in another region not anatomically related to the affected nerve.
Pain Perception	Pain experience in the cortex cerebri.
Pain Reaction	The brain's reaction to pain perception.
Pain Threshold	The least experience of pain that a subject can recognize.
Pain Tolerance Level	The greatest level of pain that a subject is prepared to tolerate.
Pain Tract Printing	The brain remembers certain pain tracts when they are stimulated often.
Paraesthesia	An abnormal sensation, whether spontaneous or evoked.
Prostaglandins	Fatty acids produced as a response to inflammation, with pain producing abilities.
Substance P	Peptide responsible for pain transmission in many pain tracts as a transmitter substance.

Subject index

116

117